QuickCook

QuickCook

Party time

Recipes listed by cooking time

30

20

10

QuickCook
Recipes for Kids

Recipes by Emma Frost

Every dish, three ways – you choose!
30 minutes | 20 minutes | 10 minutes

An Hachette UK Company
www.hachette.co.uk

First published in Great Britain in 2013 by Hamlyn,
a division of Octopus Publishing Group Ltd
Endeavour House, 189 Shaftesbury Avenue
London WC2H 8JY
www.octopusbooks.co.uk
www.octopusbooksusa.com

Distributed in the US by Hachette Book Group USA
237 Park Avenue, New York NY 10017 USA

Distributed in Canada by Canadian Manda Group
165 Dufferin Street, Toronto, Ontario, Canada M6K 3H6

ISBN 978-0-600-62526-1

Printed and bound in China

10 9 8 7 6 5 4 3 2 1

Standard level spoon and cup measurements are used in all recipesl

Ovens should be preheated to the specified temperature. If using a convection oven,
follow the manufacturer's instructions for adjusting the time and temperature.
Broilers should also be preheated.

This book includes dishes made with nuts and nut derivatives. It is advisable for
those with known allergic reactions to nuts and nut derivatives and those who may
be potentially vulnerable to these allergies, such as pregnant and nursing mothers,
people with weakened immune systems, the elderly, babies, and children, to avoid
dishes made with nuts and nut oils.

It is also prudent to check the labels of prepared ingredients for the possible inclusion
of nut derivatives.

The U.S. Food and Drug Administration advises that eggs should not be consumed
raw. This book contains some dishes made with raw or lightly cooked eggs. It is
prudent for more vulnerable people, such as pregnant and nursing mothers, people
with weakened immune systems, the elderly, babies, and young children, to avoid
uncooked or lightly cooked dishes made with eggs.

Contents

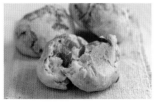
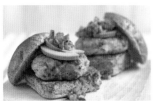
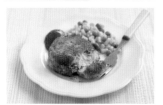
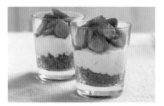
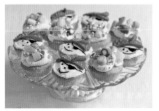

Introduction

30 20 10—Quick, Quicker, Quickest

This book offers a new and flexible approach to planning meals for busy cooks, letting you choose the recipe option that best fits the time you have available. Inside you will find 360 dishes that will inspire and motivate you to get cooking every day of the year. All the recipes take a maximum of 30 minutes to cook. Some take as little as 20 minutes and, amazingly, many take only 10 minutes. With a little preparation, you can easily try out one new recipe from this book each night and slowly you will be able to build a wide and exciting portfolio of recipes to suit your needs.

How Does it Work?

Every recipe in the QuickCook series can be cooked one of three ways—a 30-minute version, a 20-minute version, or a superquick-and-easy 10-minute version. At the beginning of each chapter you'll find recipes listed by time. Choose a dish based on how much time you have and turn to that page.

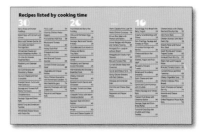

You'll find the main recipe in the middle of the page accompanied by a beautiful photograph, as well as two time-variation recipes below.

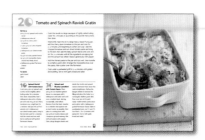

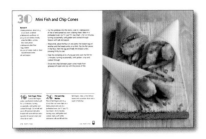

If you enjoy your chosen dish, why not go back and cook the other time-variation options at a later date? So, if you liked the 20-minute Fish and Chip Rolls, but only have 10 minutes to spare this time around, you'll find a way to cook it using quick ingredients or clever shortcuts.

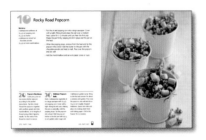

If you love the ingredients and flavors of the 10-minute Rocky Road Popcorn, why not try something more substantial, such as the 20-minute Popcorn Necklaces, or be inspired to make a more elaborate version, like the 30-minute Malt Ball and Popcorn Balls? Alternatively, browse through all 360 delicious recipes, find something that catches your eye, then cook the version that fits your time frame.

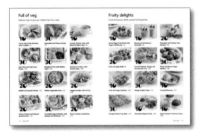

Or, for easy inspiration, turn to the gallery on pages 12–19 to get an instant overview by themes, such as Fruity delights or Classic crowd-pleasers.

QuickCook online

To make life easier, you can use the special code on each recipe page to e-mail yourself a recipe card for printing, or e-mail a text-only shopping list to your phone. Go to www.hamlynquickcook.com and enter the recipe code at the bottom of each page.

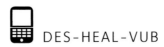

DES-HEAL-VUB

QuickCook Recipes for Kids

Cooking for our families in today's hectic times can be hard. Life is busy as we find more and more after-school activities have to be woven into our children's week. As a result, although many of us crave spending quality time together over a leisurely family meal, it often seems like there is barely enough time to eat a meal, let alone shop for it, prepare it, and cook it!

Designed for busy parents in a hurry, this book includes 100 great recipes for kids of all ages that can be cooked in 30 minutes or less. Whether you have 30, 20, or even as few as 10 minutes available, you'll find a tasty and nutritious recipe that will suit your children's taste buds as well as fit in with your busy lives. And because children can get bored with a small repertoire, there are two variations on each recipe that can be cooked in slightly less or more time.

Can good food be fast food?

This book is simple and realistic, and the recipes are genuinely fast! It is assumed you are on your own with up to four children to cook for, and that sometimes you will have to "cheat." There are some prepared ingredients in the recipes—store-bought sauces, packages of flavored grains, such as rice and couscous, and pastes, such as garlic, lemon grass, and ginger (the latter available in gourmet or Asian stores)—to add instant and intense flavors to your cooking. It is also assumed that you own a few key kitchen gadgets, such as an electric mixer, a small food processor, and a microwave. These will save you time and enable you to experiment with many different ingredients and flavors.

Another important factor in cooking well for kids is preparation. It's difficult to find the time to sit down at the beginning of the week and plan meals for the days ahead, but it helps stress levels and the household budget if you know roughly what you are going to cook. Scanning a recipe in advance will help you be sure that you have the necessary fresh, dried, and canned ingredients on hand.

For those moments when you discover you need to come up with a tasty, nutritious meal in minutes, always keep certain basic ingredients in the kitchen. Here are some suggestions:

- all-purpose flour and cornstarch
- dried pasta shapes, rice, and couscous
- quick protein, such as tuna, cheese, shrimp, and chicken
- all types of canned beans
- intense flavorings, such as bouillon cubes, soy sauce, dried herbs and spices (especially cumin, coriander, cinnamon, mixed herbs, and nutmeg)
- cans of tomatoes and coconut milk
- jars of olives, pesto, and pastes such as garlic and ginger
- frozen vegetables, such as chopped spinach, peas, and corn kernels, frozen fruit, such as raspberries.

It's also a good idea to buy in some vital "quick" ingredients for those days when time is really stretched. Ready-to-bake rolled pie dough crust and puff pastry, cooked chicken, pita breads, vanilla pudding powder, prepared pizza pie crusts and crescent roll dough, cooked rice and mashed potatoes, and cans of condensed soups are just some of the "instant" ingredients used in the recipes.

Fast and healthy!

Being in a hurry does not mean compromising on nutritional value. Getting kids used to healthy food means they are will be less likely to crave bad food as they enter their teens and gives them a much better chance of growing into fit and healthy adults.

Simple changes to your buying and cooking habits will give your children the best start. One small but significant change is to cut out salt from your cooking (officially known as sodium); this is a vital mineral that helps with muscular movement, messages to the nerves, and the pH of blood. However, it is not necessary to add it to your cooking. It is found naturally in every type of food and is especially high in processed foods. Salt is a taste we learn to expect; if you eradicate it from your cooking while your children are young, they quickly become used to the flavors of food without it.

Other small changes you can make include replacing canned fruits with fresh, limiting processed meats, such as bacon, sausages, and ham to no more than 2–3 times per week, and substituting refined white flour products, such as bread, pasta, and wraps with whole-wheat versions.

Whole grains will give your child slow-release energy and a host of nutrients not found in the refined versions; however, these foods have a slightly nuttier, denser flavor and take a little getting used to. Persist with the changes and your children will benefit.

Dealing with the fussy eater

The frustration felt by a parent of a fussy eater is immense; you want so much to feed your children wholesome, tasty, attractive meals. You work hard to create breakfasts, lunches, snacks, and dinners that all the children will eat and enjoy, but preparing a meal that is instantly rejected is very disheartening.

You can tackle the problem in a number of ways. First, make the child hungry! A fussy eater who is known for rejecting vegetables, and who has been snacking on candies or potato chips since they got home from school, is unlikely to dive into a bowl of vegetarian chili at 6 p.m. with enthusiasm. Fussy eaters need snacks, but be sure they are healthy and are eaten with at least 2 hours to spare before the next meal. If your child is hungry before dinner is ready, put out a bowl of hummus and vegetable sticks. A genuinely hungry child will eat.

Second, get the fussy eater involved with their meal. From a young age, most kids love to cook, but we forget this as they grow up. Time pressures mean we often keep the kitchen door shut when preparing meals to save ourselves from interruptions. Remember, your children can help you! If they want to get involved and time is not on your side, give them some easy jobs, such as sifting the flour or cutting out the pastry dough circles for the mini quiches (page 66). Alternatively, get them dipping chicken strips into couscous (page 56) or cracking eggs into a bowl. If they feel involved, they are less likely to reject the end result.

Third, instead of serving a prepared meal on individual plates, let the children help themselves from a large serving bowl of food in the middle of the table. A fussy eater likes to think he or she has chosen his or her own meal—give the child choice, within reason, and let the fussy eater feel in control.

Finally, many children today are unaware of where their food comes from. Put food into its context by visiting farms and food producers and making your children aware of what goes into making the food they are eating. If you can get into the countryside, let your kids pick their own fruit, so they know what is in season and when. Or if you can't make it to a farm, then buy peas in their shells and shell them together at the table. If you have a small patch of ground in the yard, or even a windowsill, a fun thing to do is to grow some produce at home. Zucchini, potatoes, carrots, tomatoes, and certain herbs are all easy to grow. Kids love the outdoors; if they equate fruit and vegetables with the outdoor activities of sowing, growing, and picking, they are much more likely to enjoy eating them.

Patience in a hurry
Fussy children, stressed parents, and a lack of time are rarely a good combination, but this book offers you more than 300 delicious, quick, and easy recipes that will fit your family's tastes, timings, and budget. Set aside a few minutes today to choose the meals that you think will work for your kids, order your shopping online, and then among the chaos of school pickups and drop-offs, baseball training, and music recitals, you will at least know that the food for next week is already taken care of!

Full of veg

Delicious ways to give your children their five-a-day!

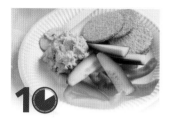

Carrot and Cumin Hummus with Crudités 42

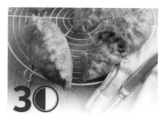

Vegetable and Cheese Turnovers 70

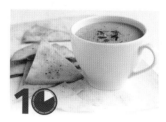

Creamy Tomato Soup with Baked Tortilla Chips 96

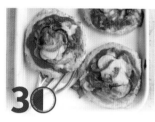

Easy Ham and Vegetable Pizzas 100

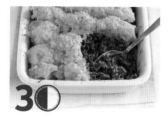

Lamb Casserole (with Hidden Veg!) 104

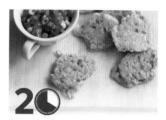

Corn Fritters with Tomato Salsa 108

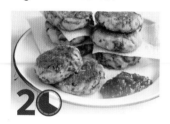

Potato and Cabbage Patties 116

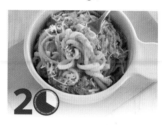

Hidden Vegetable Pasta 120

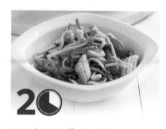

Veggie Noodles with Hoisin Sauce 126

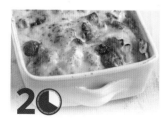

Cherry Tomato and Spinach Ravioli Gratin 130

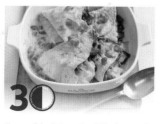

Scrambled Egg Enchiladas with Spinach and Tomatoes 164

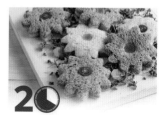

Flower Garden Sandwiches 272

Fruity delights

Sweet and savory dishes, packed full of goodness.

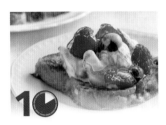

Spiced French Fruit Bread with Yogurt and Berries 24

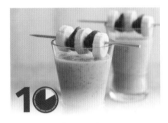

Banana and Strawberry Smoothie 38

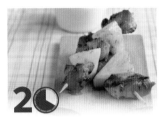

Pineapple and Chunky Ham Skewers 64

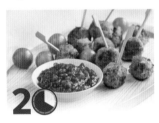

Pork and Apple Balls 84

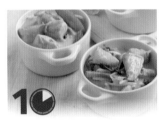

Curried Chicken, Mango, and Coconut Stir-Fry 142

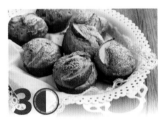

Peach and Brown Sugar Muffins 198

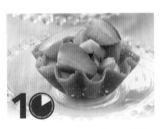

Fruit and Yogurt Baskets 206

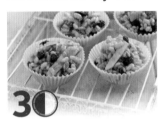

Mango Krispie Cakes 212

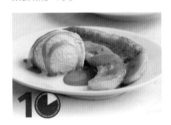

Caramel Bananas 214

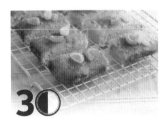

Orange Drizzle Sheet Cake 226

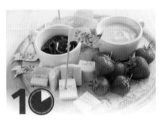

Chocolate Dipped Fruits 230

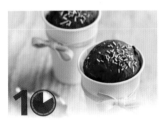

Quick Summer Fruit Ice Cream 238

Classic crowd-pleasers

Comfort food and familar favorites to make for the masses.

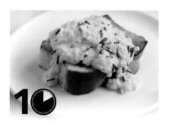

Creamy Scrambled Egg with Chives 26

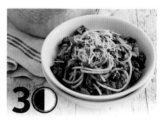

Spaghetti with Meat Sauce 134

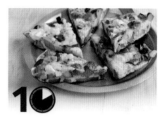

Frankfurter and Zucchini Frittata 136

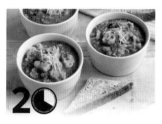

Hearty Bean, Bacon, and Pasta Soup 148

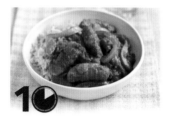

Sausage, Tomato, and Bell Pepper Pan-Fry 190

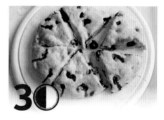

Blueberry Scones 200

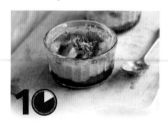

Rice Pudding and Jam Brûlée 216

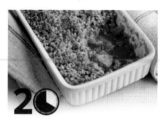

Rhubarb and Strawberry Oat Crisp 218

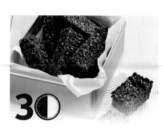

Chocolate Oat Bars 236

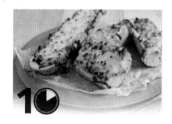

Cheesy Garlic Bread 266

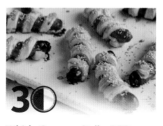

Whirly Sausage Rolls 268

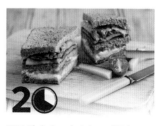

BLT Club Sandwiches 274

Give it a go

Some clever snacks, meals, and desserts for tempting those taste buds.

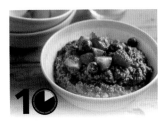
1
Chocolate Oatmeal
with Berries 30

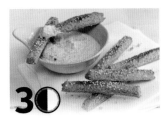
3
Whole-Wheat Cheese Straws
with Pesto Dip 52

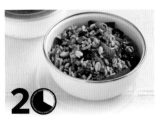
2
Brown Rice Salad with Peanuts
and Raisins 58

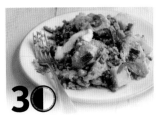
3
Curried Chicken
Couscous Salad 68

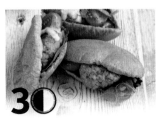
3
Mini Falafel Burgers 74

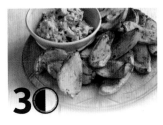
3
Potato Skins with
Guacamole 128

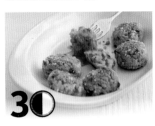
3
Spiced Rice and Chickpea Balls
with Sweet Chili Sauce 156

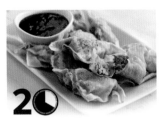
2
Pork Dumplings with
Dipping Sauce 178

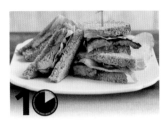
1
Curried Lamb Steak
Sandwiches 184

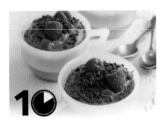
1
Chocolate Desserts with
Hidden Prunes 204

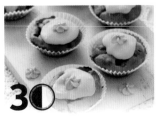
3
Iced Banana and
Raspberry Buns 232

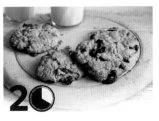
2
Spiced Raisin and
Cranberry Cookies 240

Chicken favorites

Protein-packed and full of flavor, great chicken dishes for everyday eating.

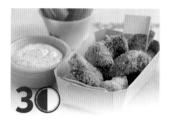

Crunchy Chicken Pesto Dippers 56

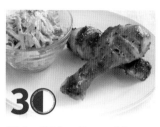

Sticky Chicken Drumsticks with Homemade Coleslaw 72

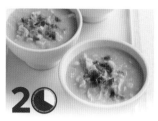

Chicken and Corn Soup 86

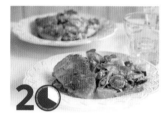

Parmesan Chicken Salad 94

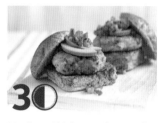

Mexican Chicken and Avocado Burgers with Salsa 98

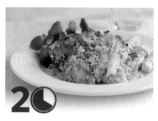

Creamy Chicken and Broccoli Pasta Gratin 102

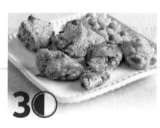

Chicken Nuggets with Sun-Dried Tomato Sauce 122

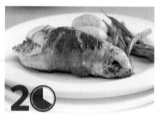

Chicken, Pesto, and Bacon Pan-Fry 132

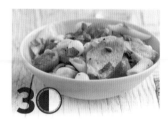

Warm Mozzarella, Chicken, Tomato, and Basil Pasta 152

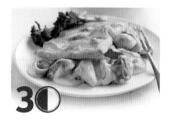

Chicken, Bacon, and Leek Pies 174

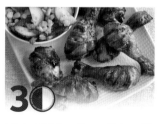

Sticky Chicken Drumsticks with Cucumber and Corn 182

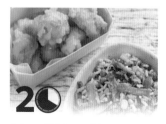

Crispy Chicken with Egg-Fried Rice 188

Fish favorites

Fried, in a casserole, stir-fried, or served in a wrap, these are great for fish fans.

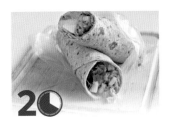

Tuna and Corn Wraps 50

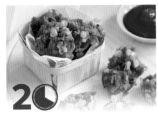

Tuna and Corn Nuggets 90

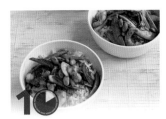

Sweet Chili Shrimp and Green Vegetable Stir-Fry 92

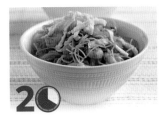

Singapore Noodles 110

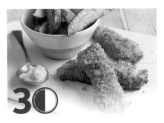

Fish Sticks with Sweet Potato Fries 112

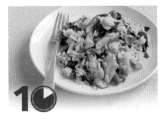

Kedgeree-Style Rice with Spinach 150

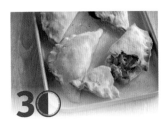

Tuna, Bell Pepper, and Cheese Calzone 162

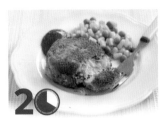

Salmon and Broccoli Fish Cakes 168

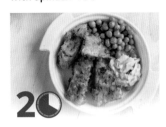

Lemon Cod Strips with Caperless Tartar Sauce 172

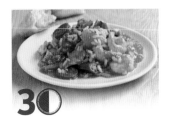

Chorizo, Chicken, and Shrimp Jambalaya 176

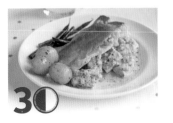

Creamy Pesto Fish Casserole 180

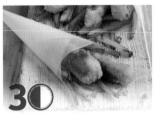

Mini Fish and Chip Cones 276

Food fun

Finger food and tasty treats to brighten up any table. Girls and boys will love these!

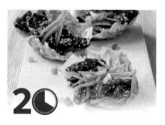

**Honeyed Duck Strips in
Lettuce "Boats"** 62

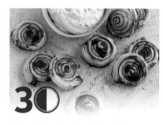

**Marmite Pinwheels with
Cream Cheese Dip** 76

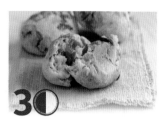

**Pepperoni and
Bell Pepper Rolls** 78

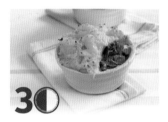

**Creamy Pork and
Apple Pies** 154

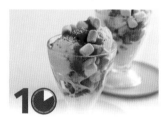

**Strawberry Ice Cream
Sundae** 210

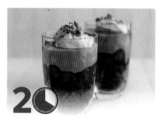

Chocolate Muffin Trifles 244

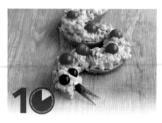

Slippery Snake 250

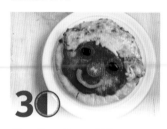

Pizza Bear Faces 252

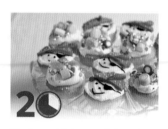

Pirate and Princess Cakes 256

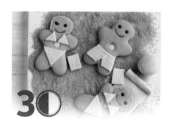

**Gingerbread People
Beach Party** 258

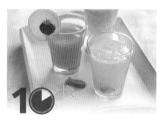

Mocktails 260

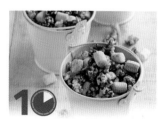

Rocky Road Popcorn 270

Weekend treats

Delicious food for cooking and enjoying together as a family.

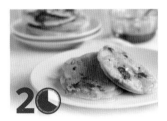

Raspberry and Oatmeal Pancakes with Syrup 36

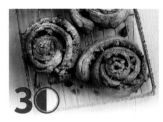

Cinnamon Buns 46

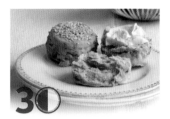

Ricotta and Tomato Biscuits 60

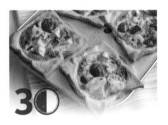

Mini Brie and Tomato Quiches 66

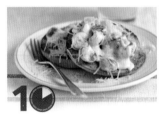

Creamy Garlic Mushroom Bagels 118

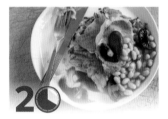

Hash Browns with Bacon and Mushrooms 146

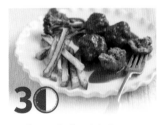

Beef Meatballs with Gravy and Baked Fries 166

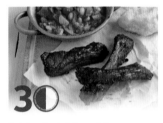

Sticky Pork Ribs with Homemade Baked Beans 186

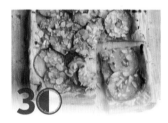

Apple and Almond Tart 222

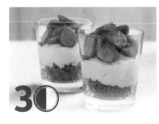

Strawberry and Lime Cheesecakes 224

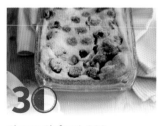

Cherry Clafouti 228

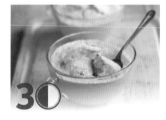

Saucy Lemon Desserts 234

QuickCook

Breakfast
& Lunchbox

Recipes listed by cooking time

10

10 Spiced French Fruit Bread with Berry Yogurt

Serves 4

2 eggs
2 tablespoons granulated sugar
½ teaspoon ground cinnamon
¼ cup milk
2 tablespoons butter
4 slices of fruit bread
1 cup (mixed berries
½ cup Greek yogurt
4 teaspoons honey, to serve

- Beat the eggs in a bowl with the sugar, cinnamon, and milk. Heat the butter in a large, heavy skillet. Dip the fruit bread slices, 2 at a time, into the egg mixture, covering both sides, then lift into the hot skillet and cook for 1–2 minutes on each side, until golden. Repeat with the remaining fruit bread slices.

- Mix half the berries into the yogurt.

- Serve the warm fruit bread slices with spoonfuls of the fruit yogurt, sprinkled with the remaining berries and drizzled with the honey.

---

20 Fruit Bread and Berry Pan Pudding

Tear 4 slices of fruit bread into bite-size pieces. Put 2 eggs, 2 tablespoons granulated sugar, ½ teaspoon ground cinnamon, and ⅔ cup milk into a bowl and mix well. Add the bread to the bowl and set aside to soak up the milk for 5 minutes. Heat 2 tablespoons butter in a medium ovenproof skillet and pour in the bread and milk mixture. Sprinkle with ½ cup mixed berries. Cook over medium heat for 3–4 minutes, until the bottom is set. Place the skillet under a preheated medium broiler (keeping the handle away from the heat) and cook for 4–5 minutes, until the top is set. Serve warm spooned into serving bowls with yogurt for a warming breakfast or dessert.

30 Berry Bread and Butter Puddings

Spread 6 slices of fruit bread with 2 tablespoons butter, then cut them into triangles. Place half the bread in the bottom of a lightly buttered ovenproof dish, then sprinkle with ½ cup berries. Put the remaining bread slices over the top. Mix 2 eggs with ⅔ cup milk, ½ teaspoon ground cinnamon, and 2 tablespoons grainulated sugar, then pour it over the bread slices and fruit. Bake in a preheated oven, at 350°F, for 15–20 minutes, until golden and just setting. Serve spooned into serving bowls with honey and yogurt, if desired.

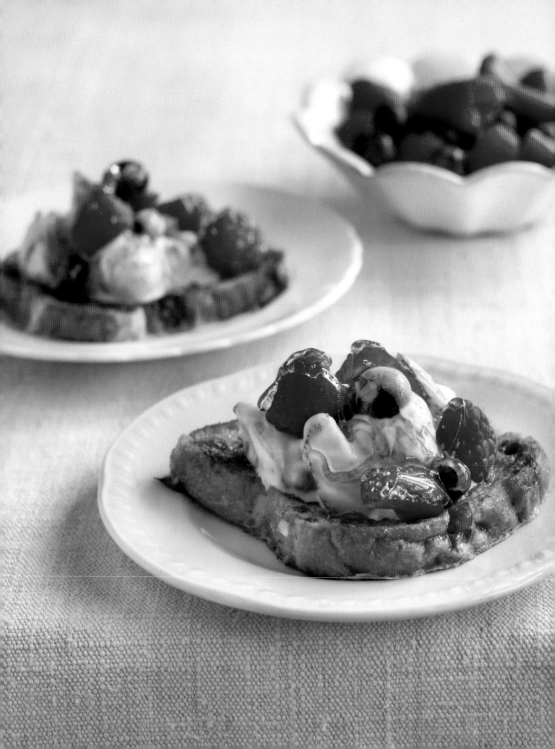

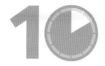

Creamy Scrambled Egg with Chives

Serves 2

2 thick slices of brioche
4 eggs
⅓ cup water
1 tablespoon butter
2 tablespoons finely grated
   Parmesan cheese
¼ cup crème fraîche or
   Greek yogurt
2 tablespoons snipped chives
black pepper

- Lightly toast the brioche slices under a preheated broiler until just golden, then turn over and lightly toast on the other side. Keep warm.

- Break the eggs into a saucepan, add the the measured water and butter, and beat together. Season generously with black pepper.

- Cook over medium heat, stirring continuously, until just beginning to scramble. Add the Parmesan and continue to cook, stirring and watching carefully, being careful to avoid overcooking the eggs, until the eggs are soft and slightly runny. Remove from the heat when almost cooked and stir in the crème fraîche or Greek yogurt and chives.

- Pile onto the warm brioche slices and serve warm with a sauce of your choice, if desired.

Chive and Parmesan Egg-Coated Brioche Mix 3 eggs in a bowl with ⅔ cup milk, 2 tablespoons Parmesan cheese, and ¼ cup chopped chives. Add 4 slices of brioche and let soak up the egg mixture for 3–4 minutes. Heat 2 tablespoons olive oil in a large, heavy skillet. Using a spatula, lift 2 of the brioche slices from the egg mixture and cook over high heat for 2 minutes on each side until golden. Repeat with the other 2 slices. Serve 2 per person, sprinkled with a little more Parmesan and chopped chives, if desired.

Baked Eggs with Spinach and Chives Lightly grease 2 ramekins with 1 tablespoon butter, add 1 tablespoon finely grated Parmesan cheese to each, and push around the ramekin to coat. Place 1 (5 oz) package washed spinach leaves in a saucepan over high heat and stir for 2–3 minutes, until wilted. Remove from the heat, put the spinach in a colander, and squeeze out any excess water. Divide between the ramekins. Break 1 egg into each of the ramekins, then top each with a pinch of grated nutmeg and 1½ teaspoons chopped chives on each. Bake in a preheated oven, at 350°F, for 15–20 minutes, until the eggs are just set. Serve with brioche slices or crusty bread.

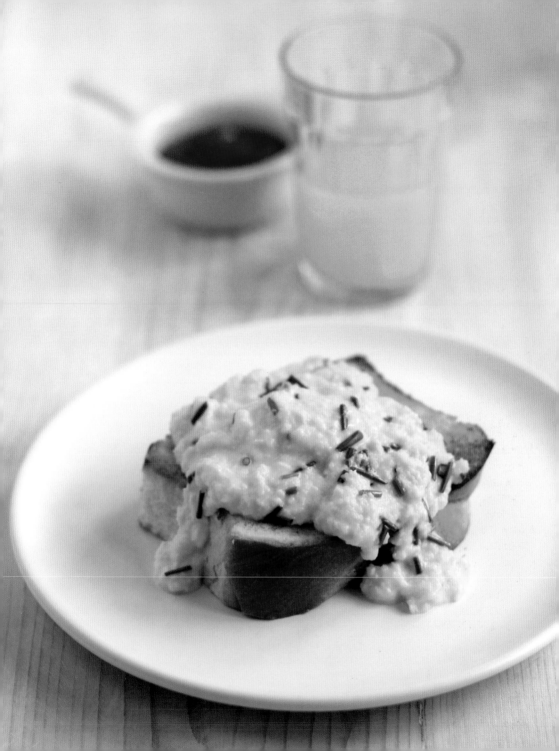

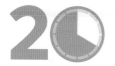

Sausage, Bacon, and Tomato Frittata

Serves 4

flour, for dusting
6 oz bulk sausage or sausage meat removed from casings
2 tablespoons olive oil
6 bacon slices, chopped
4 small tomatoes, cut into wedges
6 eggs
black pepper
¼ cup chopped parsley, to garnish
slices of toast, to serve

- Using lightly floured hands, divide the sausage meat into 8 pieces. Shape into rough balls, then lightly flatten.

- Heat the oil in a heavy, nonstick skillet. Add the sausage meat patties and cook over medium heat for 5 minutes, turning once, until golden and cooked through. Add the bacon and cook for another 3 minutes, until cooked.

- Add the tomatoes, remove from the heat, and evenly spread the ingredients around the skillet.

- Beat the eggs, then season with black pepper and pour into the skillet. Return to the heat and cook over medium heat for 3–4 minutes, until the bottom is set. Place the skillet under a preheated hot broiler (keeping the handle away from the heat) and cook for 3–4 minutes, until it is set.

- Divide into wedges and serve with slices of toast.

Pan-Fried Egg, Sausage, and Tomato on Toast
Heat 2 tablespoons olive oil in a skillet. With lightly floured hands, divide 6 oz bulk sausage or sausage meat into 8 balls; press into patties. Cook the patties in a little oil over medium heat for 4–5 minutes, turning once, until cooked, adding 4 halved small tomatoes for the final 2 minutes. In a separate nonstick skillet, heat 1 tablespoon olive oil and cook 2 eggs over medium heat for 2–3 minutes. Serve on toast.

Bacon and Tomato Quiche
Unroll 1 store-bought rolled dough pie crust and use to line a 12 x 8 inch shallow baking pan. Sprinkle 4 oz precooked bacon, broken into small pieces, and 5 small tomatoes, cut into wedges, into the pan. Beat 6 eggs with 3 tablespoons chopped parsley and plenty of black pepper in a small bowl, then pour the egg mixture over the bacon and tomato. Bake in a preheated oven, at 400°F, for 20 minutes, until well risen and golden. The quiche will sink as you remove it from the oven. Serve cut into wedges. A great breakfast to eat on the move!

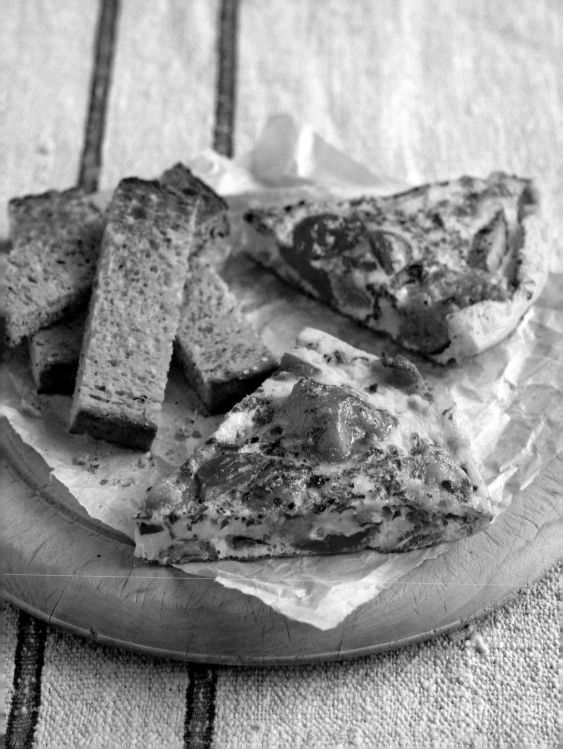

10 Chocolate Oatmeal with Berries

Serves 2

2½ cups milk (or rice milk
  for a dairy-free option)
1 cup rolled oats
3 tablespoons cocoa powder, plus
  extra for dusting (optional)
¼ cup firmly packed brown sugar
¾ cup mixed berries
2 tablespoons maple syrup

- Place the milk in a heavy saucepan with the oats and bring to a boil. Add the cocoa powder and sugar, then reduce the heat and simmer for 6–7 minutes, stirring occasionally, until the oats have swollen and the oatmeal has thickened, adding a little water to loosen, if necessary.

- Mix the berries with the maple syrup. Serve the oatmeal in warmed serving bowls with the berries spooned into the center. Dust with cocoa powder, if desired.

20 Chocolate and Fruit Muesli

Place 3 cups rolled oats in a large bowl, add 2 tablespoons cocoa powder, and toss well. Coarsely chop ½ cup toasted hazelnuts and 1 cup fresh or dried chopped dates and add to the bowl. Coarsely crumble 1 cup banana chips and toss into the mixture. Add 1 tablespoon hemp seeds and 1¼ cups bran flakes and toss again. Spoon a little of the muesli into a cereal bowl and pour milk over it to cover. Let stand for 5 minutes to let the oats swell, then add a little more milk to taste. Sprinkle with unbleached granulated sugar to serve, if desired.

30 Chocolate and Raisin Oat Bars

Place 1¼ cups boiling water in a saucepan with 1¼ cups rolled oats, ⅓ cup raisins, 3 tablespoons cocoa powder, and ¼ cup firmly packed brown sugar and bring back to a boil. Reduce the heat to a simmer and stir continuously for about 2–3 minutes, until very thick. Transfer to an 8 inch square cake pan and smooth the top. Chill for 20 minutes, until solid, then cut into 12 squares or bars to serve (these will keep for up to 3 days refrigerated in an airtight container).

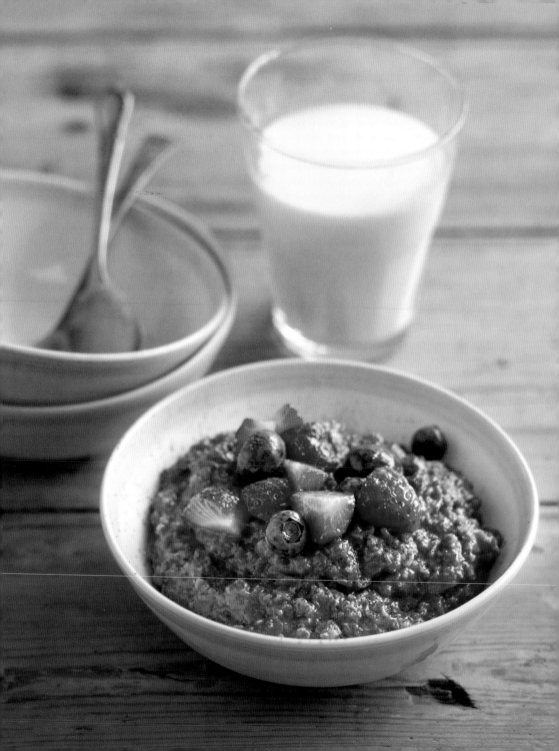

Whole-Wheat Cheese and Bacon Breakfast Muffins

Makes 12

3 cups whole-wheat flour
4 teaspoons baking powder
1 teaspoon baking soda
2 teaspoons dry mustard
1 cup shredded cheddar cheese
2 oz cooked bacon, chopped
2 eggs
¾ cup vegetable oil
1 cup milk
salt and black pepper

- Line a 12-cup muffin pan with 12 paper muffin liners.

- Sift the flour, baking powder, baking soda, and dry mustard into a bowl and season with a pinch of salt and black pepper. Stir in the cheese and bacon pieces.

- Mix together the egg with the oil and milk in a small bowl, then pour into the dry ingredients and mix well, adding a little milk if the batter is too dry.

- Divide the batter evenly among the paper liners and bake in a preheated oven, at 350°F, for 20–25 minutes, until golden and risen.

- Serve warm, if possible, but they are equally delicious cold.

 Cheese and Bacon Griddle Biscuits

Place 2 cups whole-wheat flour in a bowl with 2 teaspoons baking powder, a pinch of salt, ¼ cup shredded cheddar cheese, 1 oz finely broken cooked bacon pieces, 1 egg, and 1 cup milk and mix well. Brush a skillet with a little melted butter. Drop small mounds of the batter from a spoon or small ladle into the skillet and cook over medium heat for 2 minutes, then turn the biscuits over with a spatula and cook for another 1–2 minutes, until golden. Repeat with the remaining batter. Serve warm.

 Cheese and Bacon Sheet Cake

Place 2 cups whole-wheat flour in a bowl with 1 tablespoon baking powder and 1 teaspoon dry mustard. Mix in ¾ cup shredded cheddar cheese and 2 oz chopped cooked bacon pieces and stir well. Beat 1 egg with ¼ cup vegetable oil and ¼ cup milk in a small bowl, then pour into the dry ingredients and mix well. Pour into a well-greased 7 x 11 inch jelly roll pan and bake in a preheated oven, at 350°F, for 12–15 minutes, until well risen and golden.

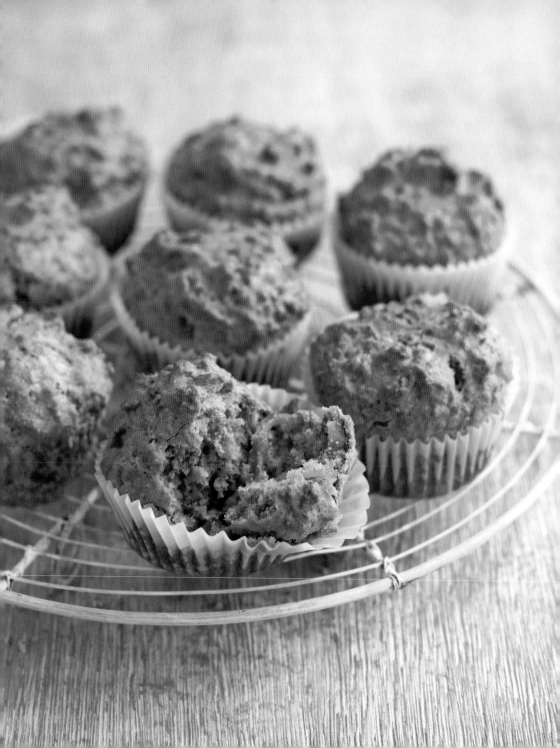

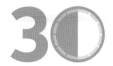

On-the-Go Granola Breakfast Bars

Makes 9

6 tablespoons butter, plus extra for greasing

¾ cup honey

½ teaspoon ground cinnamon

¾ cup coarsely chopped dried apricots

½ cup coarsely chopped dried papaya or mango

⅓ cup raisins

¼ cup mixed seeds, such as pumpkin, sesame, and sunflower

½ cup coarsely chopped pecans

1⅔ cups rolled oats

- Grease a shallow 8 inch square pan.

- Place the butter and honey in a saucepan and bring to a boil, stirring continuously, until the mixture bubbles. Add the cinnamon, dried fruit, seeds, and nuts, then stir and heat for 1 minute. Remove from the heat and add the oats. Stir well, then transfer to the prepared pan and press down well. Bake in a preheated oven, at 375°F, for 15 minutes, until the top is just beginning to brown.

- Let cool in the pan, then cut into 9 squares or bars to serve.

 Granola, Yogurt, and Fruit Layer

Divide 1⅓ cups prepared granola cereal among 4 glasses and top each with ¼ cup Greek yogurt. Chop ¾ cup mixed dried fruits, such as mango, apricots, and raisins, and toss with 2 pinches of ground cinnamon. Spoon on top of the yogurt and drizzle each with 1 teaspoon honey to serve.

 Homemade Granola Cereal

Place 3 cups rolled oats in a bowl with 2 tablespoons vegetable oil, ⅓ cup honey, ½ teaspoon ground cinnamon, and 1 teaspoon vanilla extract and stir well to coat. Spread onto a baking sheet and bake in a preheated oven, at 350°F, for 10–15 minutes, until lightly golden. Stir in ½ cup chopped dried apricots, ½ cup dried papaya or mango, ½ cup raisins, and 3 tablespoons mixed seeds. Serve in bowls with milk.

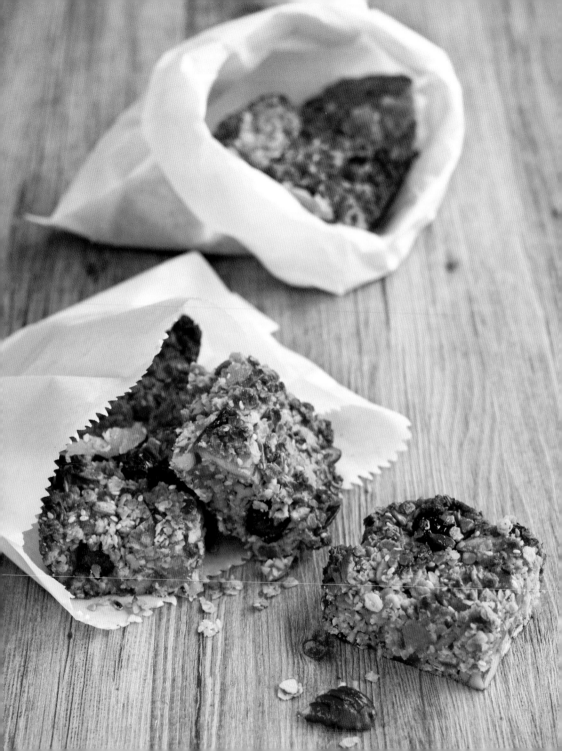

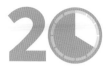

Raspberry and Oat Pancakes

Makes 8

1 cup all-purpose flour

1 teaspoon baking powder

2 tablespoons granulated sugar

2 tablespoons rolled oats

1 egg, beaten

½ teaspoon vanilla extract

⅔ cup milk

½ cup raspberries, halved

oil, for frying

½ cup maple syrup, to serve

- Place the flour in a bowl with the baking powder, sugar, and oats and stir well. Make a well in the center and set aside. Beat together the egg, vanilla extract, and milk in a small bowl, then pour into the dry ingredients and beat lightly to make a batter the consistency of thick cream. Carefully fold in the raspberries.

- Lightly oil a heavy skillet or flat griddle pan. Drop tablespoons of the batter onto the pan surface until covered, and cook over medium heat for 1–2 minutes, until bubbles rise to the surface and burst. Turn the pancakes over and cook for another 1–2 minutes, until golden and set. Remove from the pan and keep warm. Repeat with the remaining batter to make 8 pancakes.

- Serve warm, on warmed plates, with 1 tablespoon maple syrup spooned over each.

Raspberry Pancake Towers

Lightly toast 8 store-bought pancakes under a preheated hot broiler for 1–2 minutes on each side until warm and pale golden. Place 1 on a warmed serving plate and top with 1 tablespoon raspberry preserves and 4–5 raspberries. Top with another warm pancake, a spoonful of Greek yogurt or vanilla-flavored yogurt, and a drizzle of maple syrup. Repeat with the remaining pancakes.

Baked Raspberry and Oatmeal

Put 1⅓ cups all-purpose flour, 1¼ teaspoons baking powder, 3 tablespoons granulated sugar, and 3 tablespoons rolled oats into a bowl. Beat 2 eggs with ½ teaspoon vanilla extract and 1 cup milk, then add to the dry ingredients and beat well. Pour into a well-greased shallow ovenproof dish and sprinkle with 1¼ cups raspberries. Mix 2 tablespoons granulated sugar with ½ teaspoon ground cinnamon and sprinkle over the top. Bake in a preheated oven, at 400°F, for 20 minutes, until well risen and golden. Serve warm as a delicious breakfast with spoonfuls of Greek yogurt or vanilla-flavoered yogurt, if desired.

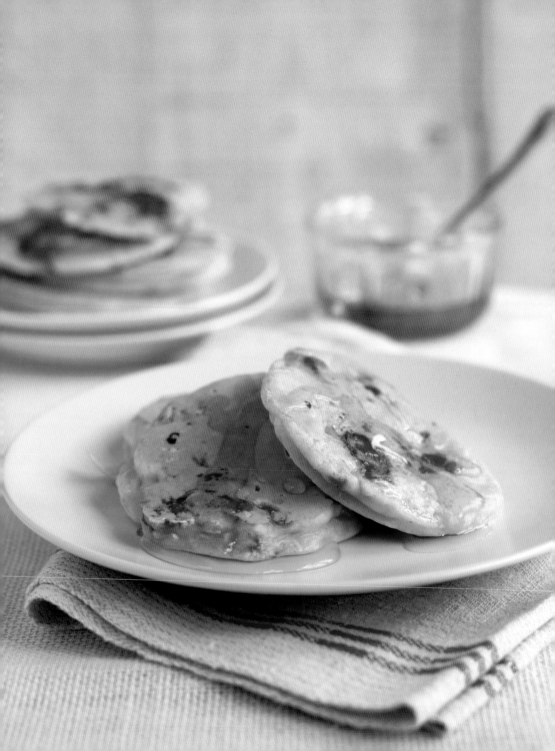

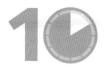 # Banana and Strawberry Smoothie

Serves 4

2 ripe bananas, coarsely chopped
½ pint strawberries, hulled
1¼ cups water
¼ cup Greek yogurt or
plain yogurt
2 tablespoons maple syrup

To serve

banana slices
strawberry halves

- Place the bananas in a food processor with the strawberries and milk. Process until almost smooth. Add the yogurt and maple syrup and give another short blast of the food processor to mix.

- Pour into 4 small glasses and decorate each with a toothpick threaded with banana slices and strawberry halves for the children to dip.

Warm Banana and Strawberry Breakfast Whips

Heat 1 tablespoon butter in a large, heavy skillet and cook 2 coarsely chopped bananas for 4 minutes, until warm and golden. Add 6 strawberries, hulled and coarsely chopped, and cook for 1 minute. Add 2 tablespoons maple syrup and toss, then cook for another 1 minute. Serve spooned into 4 bowls, each topped with ¼ cup Greek yogurt or vanilla-flavored yogurt. Sprinkle with a little muesli, if desired.

Ice-Cold Banana and Strawberry Shakes

Put 2 bananas into a food processor with 1¼ cups milk and ½ pint hulled strawberries and blend until smooth. Add 12 ice cubes and process again until the ice is crushed finely within the shake. Pour into a shallow container and freeze for 15 minutes, until thicker. Pour into glasses and decorate with toothpicks threaded with colorful fruit pieces of your choice.

KID-BREA-DAM

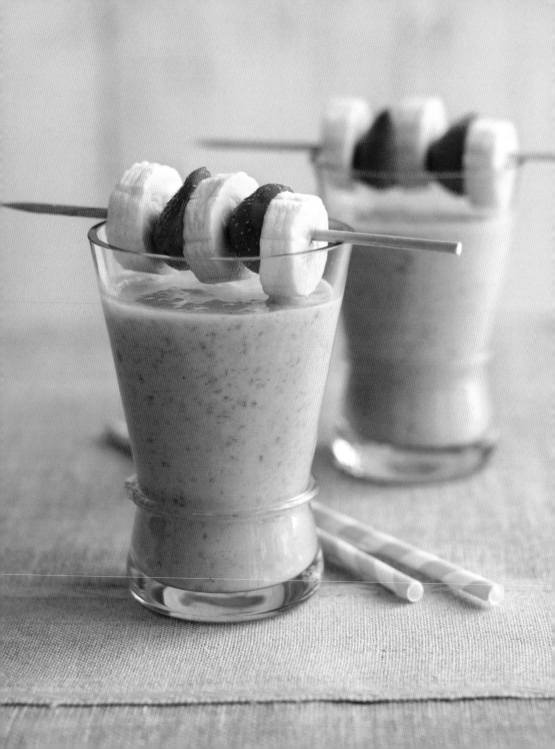

30 Cheese and Ham Croissants

Makes 6

butter, for greasing
1 (8 oz) can crescent rolls dough
12 slices of wafer-thin ham
6 thin slices of Swiss cheese
1 tablespoon Dijon mustard
beaten egg, to glaze
1 tablespoon grated Parmesan
   cheese

- Lightly grease 2 baking sheets.

- Tear the crescent roll dough along the perforations. For each croissant, unroll and lay 2 slices of ham on top of the dough, trying to keep the ham within the dough's outline, then lay 1 cheese slice over the top (this needs to be thin to be able to roll). Lightly spread with the mustard.

- Roll up the croissants, gently curl into a crescent shape, and place on the baking sheets. Brush with beaten egg, then sprinkle with the Parmesan.

- Bake in a preheated oven, at 400°F, for 10–15 minutes, until well risen and golden. Serve warm.

Quick Cheese and Ham Croissants

Cut 4 prepared croissants in half horizontally. Fill each with 2 slices of wafer-thin ham, 1 thin slice of Swiss cheese, and 2 thick tomato slices. Place on a baking sheet and bake in a preheated oven, at 400°F, for 5 minutes, until warm, then serve.

Cheesy Croissant Pinwheels

Place 1 (8 oz) can crescent roll dough on a cutting board. Using a sharp knife, cut the dough into fifteen ½ inch thick pinwheels and place on a lightly greased baking sheet, cut side up. Brush each with a little beaten egg, then sprinkle with 3 tablespoons grated Parmesan cheese. Bake in a preheated oven, at 400°F, for 10–15 minutes, until golden and lightly puffed. Serve warm with ketchup for dipping.

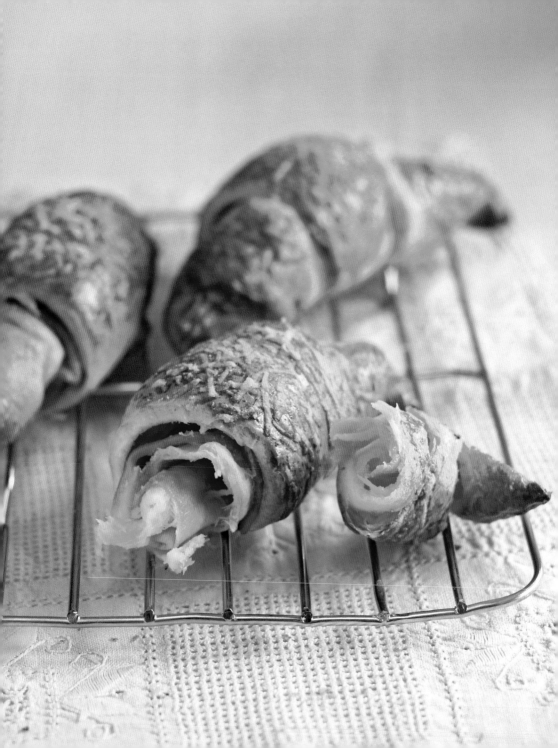

10 Carrot and Cumin Hummus with Crudités

Serves 4

4 carrots, peeled and coarsely
  chopped into bite-size pieces
1 tablespoon cumin seeds
3 tablespoons olive oil
1 (15 oz) can chickpeas,
  rinsed and drained
¼ cup tahini paste
1 teaspoon ground coriander
salt and black pepper

To serve

oat cakes, rice cakes, or toasted
  pita breads (optional)
cucumber sticks
red bell pepper slices

- Put the carrots into a skillet with the cumin seeds and oil and cook over high heat for 5 minutes, until the carrots have turned golden in places, without burning the seeds.

- Remove from the heat and place in a food processor with the chickpeas, tahini paste, and coriander. Season well with salt and black pepper and process until smooth, adding a little cold water to loosen, if necessary. Transfer to a serving bowl.

- Serve with red bell pepper slices and cucumber sticks, and oat cakes, rice cakes, or pita breads, if desired.

20 Roasted Cumin Carrots and Chickpeas

Place 6 peeled and coarsely chopped carrots in a baking pan with ¼ cup olive oil and 1 tablespoon cumin seeds and toss to coat the carrots in the seeds. Add 1 (15 oz) can chickpeas, rinsed and drained, sprinkle 2 tablespoons sesame seeds over the carrots, and roast at the top of a preheated oven, at 400°F, for 15 minutes, until hot. Serve with crusty bread.

30 Roasted Carrot, Cumin, and Feta Couscous

Place 6 peeled and chopped carrots in a baking pan with ¼ cup olive oil and 1 tablespoon cumin seeds and toss well. Roast in a preheated oven, at 400°F, for 15 minutes, until the carrots are pale golden in places. Put ¾ cup couscous in a mixing bowl, cover with hot water, and set aside for 15 minutes to swell. Meanwhile, crumble 1⅓ cups feta cheese into a serving bowl, add ¼ coarsely chopped cucumber, and mix with 1 teaspoon ground coriander. Add the swollen couscous and roasted carrots, toss together, and serve.

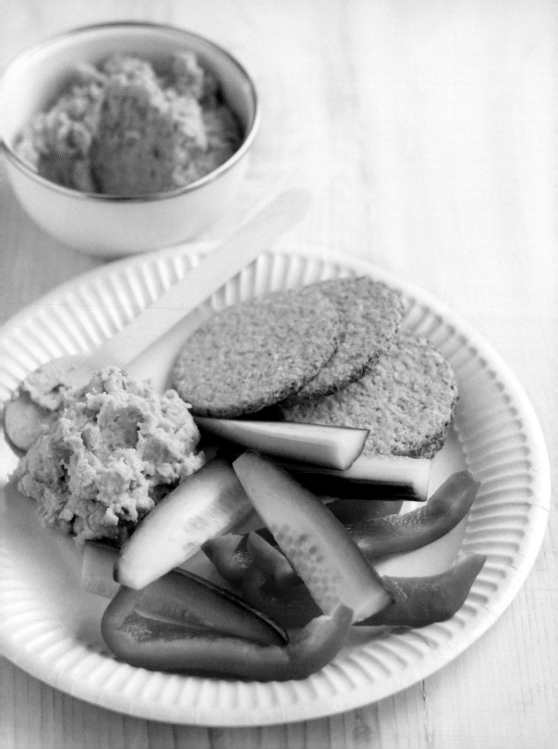

30 Sausage and Tomato Puff Pastry Turnover

Makes 4

1 sheet ready-to-bake puff
   pastry
8 oz bulk sausage or sausage
   meat removed from the casings
1 tablespoon whole-grain mustard
1 tablespoon chopped parsley
flour, for dusting
4 slices of tomato
beaten egg, to glaze
baked beans, to serve (optional)

- Unroll the pastry and cut into 4 equal rectangles. Place the sausage meat in a bowl with the mustard and parsley and mix well. Using lightly floured hands, divide the sausage meat into 4 pieces, then shape each into a rough square.

- Place 1 square at an angle in the center of 1 pastry rectangle, then place a tomato slice on top. Fold the corners of the pastry up and over the sausage meat to form an envelope shape. Place on a baking sheet and brush with beaten egg. Repeat with the remaining ingredients to make 4 turnovers.

- Bake in a preheated oven, at 400°F, for 15–20 minutes, until well risen and golden. Serve warm with hot baked beans, if desired.

 Cheesy Sausage and Tomato Rolls

Place 4 cooked sausage rolls on a baking sheet. Lay a slice of tomato on top of each and sprinkle each with 1 teaspoon grated Parmesan cheese. Bake in a preheated oven, at 400°F, for 8 minutes, until hot. Serve with hot baked beans, if desired.

 Sausage, Tomato, and Bean Puffs

Unroll 1 sheet ready-to-bake puff pastry, cut into 4 equal rectangles, and place on a baking sheet. Prick all over with a fork, then brush with beaten egg. Bake in a preheated oven, at 400°F, for 10–12 minutes, until golden and well puffed. Meanwhile heat 1 tablespoon oil in a skillet and cook 4 Vienna sausages or other small sausages for 8–10 minutes, until golden and cooked through. Add 4 small tomato halves, cut side down, for the final 3–4 minutes of cooking to soften and warm. Heat 1 (15 oz) can baked beans in a separate saucepan for 2–3 minutes, until hot, stirring occasionally. Serve the warm pastry rectangles on a plate, each piled with 1 sausage, 1 tomato half, and beans.

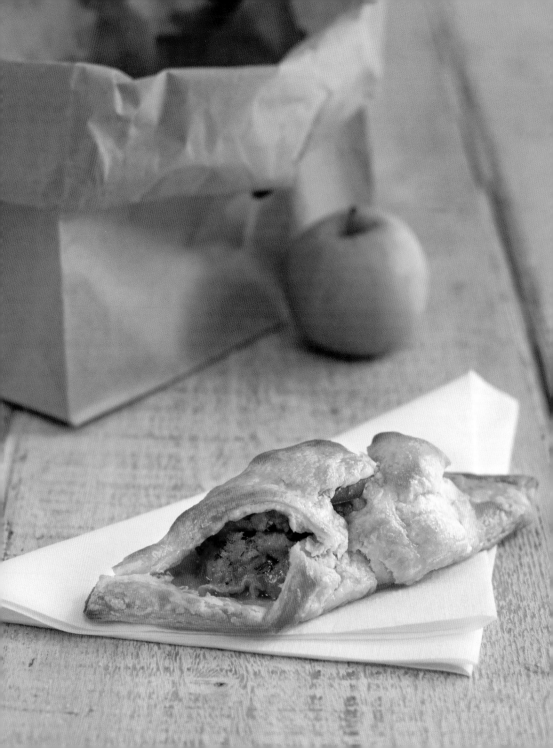

30 Cinnamon Buns

Makes 8

4 tablespoons softened butter, plus extra for greasing
1 (8 oz) can crescent roll dough
⅓ cup firmly packed brown sugar
3 teaspoons ground cinnamon
¾ cup coarsely chopped pecans (optional)
2 tablespoons confectioners' sugar, for dusting

- Lightly grease 2 baking sheets.

- Unroll the crescent roll dough on a cutting board. Place the butter, sugar, and cinnamon in a bowl and beat well with a wooden spoon until soft and well blended. Spread the cinnamon butter evenly over the dough, right to the edges. Sprinkle with the chopped pecans, if using, then tightly roll up the dough.

- Cut the log into 4 thick pinwheels and place well apart on the prepared baking sheets. Bake in a preheated oven, at 400°F, for 15–20 minutes, until well risen and golden. Serve warm, dusted with confectioners' sugar.

---

1 Toasted Fruit Bread with Cinnamon Butter Cut 8 thick slices of good-quality fruit bread and cook under a preheated broiler for about 2 minutes on each side until golden and lightly toasted. Meanwhile, beat 2 tablespoons butter with 2 tablespoons firmly packed brown sugar and 1 teaspoon ground cinnamon. Spread the butter over the toasted fruit bread and serve warm with the butter melted in.

2 Croissant Twists with Warm Cinnamon Butter Unroll 1 (8 oz) can crescent roll dough on a cutting board. Cut into 8 strips across its width, twist each one several times, and place on a nonstick baking sheet. Bake in a preheated oven, at 400°F, for 15 minutes, until golden and cooked through. Meanwhile, heat 1 stick unsalted butter in a saucepan until just beginning to melt. Transfer to a bowl and beat with 1 tablespoon ground cinnamon and ⅓ cup firmly packed brown sugar until warm, soft, and light. Place in a serving bowl and serve with the warm twists to dip in or spread over.

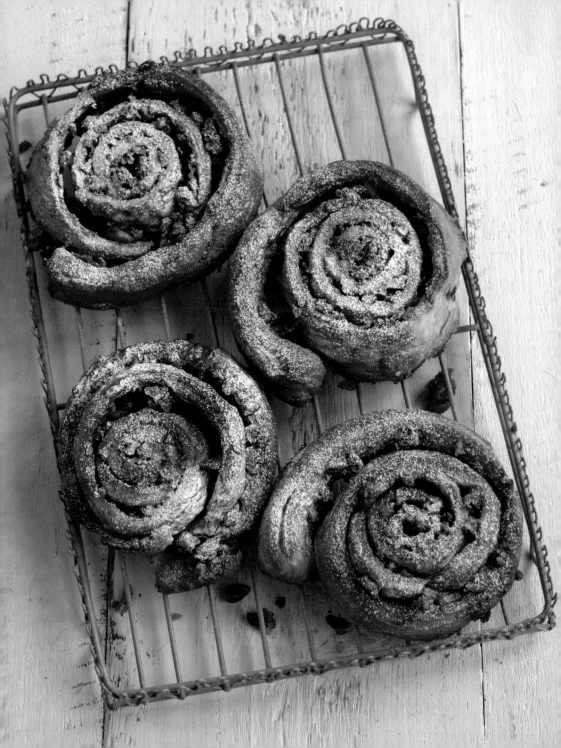

30 Sausage, Sage, and Onion Rolls

Makes 8

1 tablespoon olive oil

½ small red onion, finely chopped

1 lb bulk sausage or sausage meat removed from the casings

1 tablespoon whole-grain mustard

1 tablespoon chopped sage

1 sheet store-bought rolled dough pie crust

flour, for dusting

beaten egg, to glaze

applesauce or ketchup, to serve

- Heat the oil in a large, heavy skillet and cook the onion over medium heat for 5 minutes, until soft.

- Meanwhile, place the sausage meat in a bowl with the mustard and sage and mash together well. Add the onion and mix together.

- Unroll the dough on a floured board. Shape the sausage meat into a long sausage shape, the length of the dough, and place in the center. Lightly brush one of the long edges of the dough with beaten egg, fold the opposite edge of the dough over the sausage meat and press to seal. Using a fork, mark the edge to make sure the seal is made. Cut the long sausage roll into 8 equal pieces and place on a baking sheet. Score the tops, brush with beaten egg, and bake in a preheated oven, at 425°F, for 15 minutes, until golden and cooked. Serve with applesauce or ketchup.

 Sausage, Sage, and Onion Bread Rolls

Heat 1 tablespoon olive oil in a small skillet and cook ½ small thinly sliced red onion over medium heat for 5 minutes, until softened, stirring occasionally. Meanwhile, cook 4 small sausages under a preheated hot broiler for 8 minutes, turning frequently, until golden and cooked through. Meanwhile, carefully slice the crusts off 4 slices of whole-wheat bread. Spread one side of each bread slice with 1 tablespoon whole-grain mustard and 1 teaspoon ketchup. Sprinkle each with a pinch of dried sage, sprinkle with one-quarter of the onion, and place 1 hot sausage on top. Roll the bread tightly around the sausages and secure with toothpicks (remove the sticks before serving). Serve with applesauce or ketchup to dip.

 Sausage, Sage, and Onion Patties

Heat 1 tablespoon olive oil in a skillet and cook 1 small finely chopped red onion for 3 minutes. Transfer to a bowl, add (1 lb) sausage meat, 1 tablespoon whole-grain mustard, and 1 tablespoon chopped sage and mash to mix. Season, then stir in 1 egg yolk and ⅓ cup bread crumbs. Divide into 8, shape each piece into a ball, then press to form rounded patties. Heat 2 tablespoons olive oil in a heavy skillet and cook the patties over medium heat for 10–12 minutes, turning until golden and cooked.

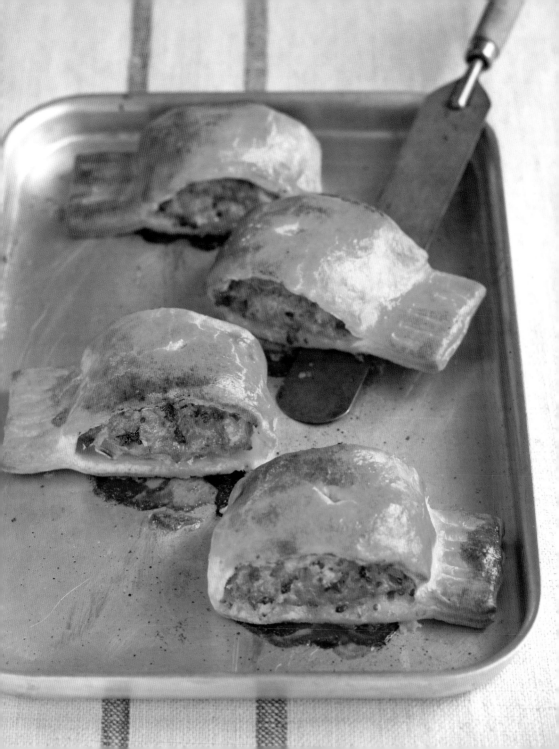

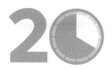 Tuna and Corn Wraps

Serves 4

2 eggs

1 (12 oz) can chunk-light tuna in water, drained

½ cup drained canned corn kernels or frozen corn kernels

¼ cup mayonnaise

4 whole-wheat flour tortillas

1 container alfalfa sprouts or other small sprouts (optional)

4 pinches of paprika

black pepper

- Place the eggs in a saucepan of water and bring to a boil. Reduce the heat and simmer for 10 minutes, until hard-boiled. Remove from the pan and plunge into cold water to cool.

- Meanwhile, place the tuna and corn kernels in a mixing bowl and season with black pepper. Add the mayonnaise and mix together.

- Lay the tortillas on a cutting board and divide the tuna mixture among them, piled across the middle of each. Shell the eggs and coarsely chop, then sprinkle over the tuna mixture. Sprinkle with the sprouts, if using. Sprinkle each with a pinch of paprika, then roll up tightly and cut in half to serve. Wrap in wax paper to travel, if desired.

---

10 Tuna and Alfalfa Sprout Dip with Crudités and Crispy Tortillas

Cut 2 tortillas into triangles and dry-fry in a skillet for 1 minute on each side until slightly crisp. Remove and set aside to cool. Place 1 (5 oz) can chunk-light tuna in water, drained, and ⅔ cup drained canned corn kernels or frozen corn kernels in a bowl with ¼ cup mayonnaise and mix well. Season with black pepper, then stir in some alfalfa sprouts and mix well. Transfer to a serving bowl and serve with sugarsnap peas and the tortillas.

30 Baked Tuna and Corn Tortillas

Mix 1 (12 oz) can chunk-light tuna in water, drained, in a bowl with 1 cup shredded cheddar cheese, ⅔ cup drained canned corn kernels or frozen corn kernels, and 4 coarsely chopped scallions. Lay 4 tortillas on a cutting board and divide the tuna mixture among them, piling onto a quarter of the area of each. Fold the tortillas into quarters to enclose the filling. Arrange in a single layer in an ovenproof dish and sprinkle with another ¾ cup shredded cheddar cheese.

Cook under a preheated medium broiler for 5–7 minutes, until the cheese has melted and the tortillas are piping hot. Serve with salad, if liked.

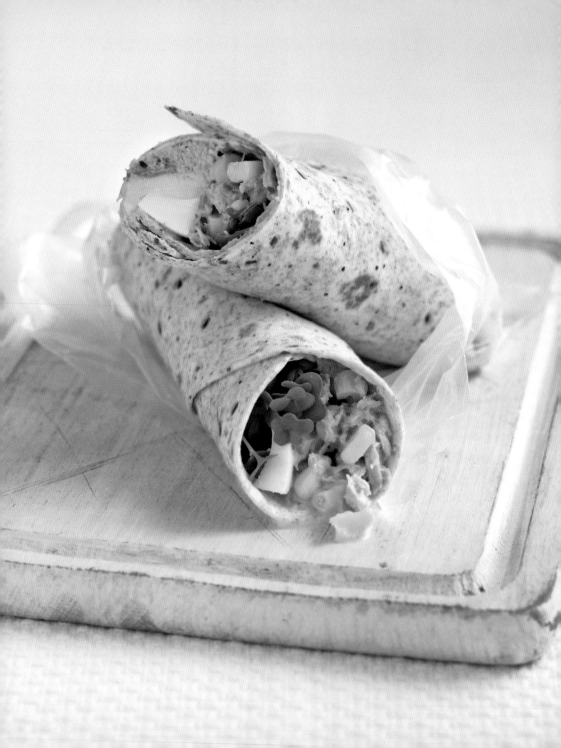

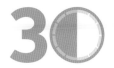

Whole-Wheat Cheese Straws with Pesto Dip

Serves 4

4 tablespoons softened butter, plus extra for greasing
1 cup shredded cheddar cheese
1 cup whole-wheat flour, plus extra for dusting
beaten egg, to glaze
2 tablespoons sesame seeds
¼ teaspoon chili powder

For the dip

3 tablespoons pesto
⅓ cup cream cheese
3 tablespoons milk

- Lightly grease a baking sheet.

- Blend the butter and cheese in a food processor. Stir in the flour and 3 tablespoons water and form into a soft dough. Turn out onto a lightly floured surface and roll out to about ¼ inch thick. Brush with beaten egg, then cut into ¾ x 4 inch long strips and sprinkle with the sesame seeds and chili powder. Place on the prepared baking sheet and bake in a preheated oven, at 400°F, for 10–15 minutes, until crisp.

- Meanwhile, make the dip. Mix the pesto with the cream cheese and milk. Place in a small dipping bowl to serve with the warm cheese straws.

 Cheese Straws with Cheesy Basil and Pine Nut Dip Put 1 cup cream cheese into a bowl with 3 tablespoons milk and blend until smooth. Coarsely chop a handful of basil and add to the cheese along with 3 tablespoons grated Parmesan cheese and 2 tablespoons coarsely chopped pine nuts. Season generously with black pepper and serve with prepared cheese straws.

 Pesto and Cheese Squares Unroll 1 sheet store-bought rolled dough pie crust on a cutting board and spread with ¼ cup pesto right to the edges. Cut into 15 squares (5 x 3) and place on a baking sheet, spaced apart. Sprinkle ½ cup finely grated Parmesan cheese over the top of each, along with 1 tablespoon sesame seeds and 1 tablespoon pumpkin seeds. Bake in a preheated oven, at 425°F, for 10–12 minutes, until golden and cooked through. Serve warm.

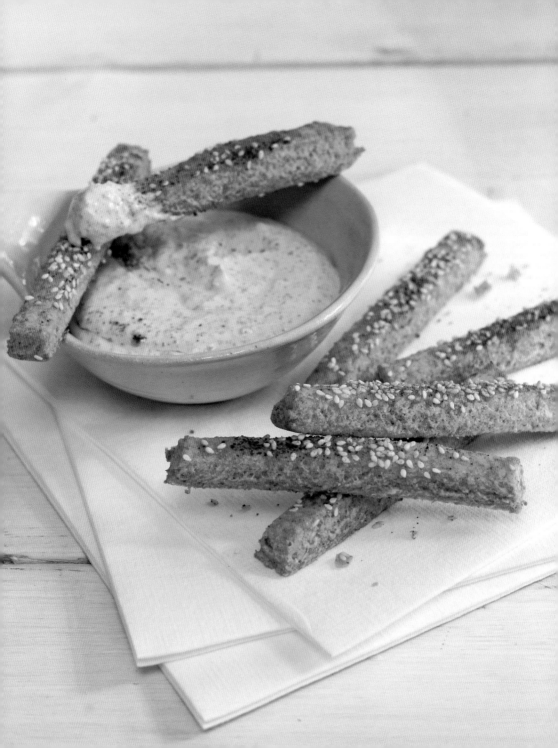

30 Picnic Loaf

Serves 6

1 large round bread loaf
4 oz salami
4 oz sliced turkey
handful of basil leaves
3 tomatoes, sliced
5 oz mozzarella cheese,
   drained and sliced
1 small red onion, cut into rings
2 handfuls of arugula
¾ cup pitted ripe black olives
3 oz cheddar cheese or
   American cheese, thinly sliced

- Cut the top off the loaf, about 1½ inches down from the top, and hollow out the inside of the loaf, pulling the soft bread out with your hands and leaving about a 1 inch edge.

- Start by layering the salami into the bottom of the hollowed-out loaf, then cover with the turkey slices. Place a layer of basil leaves on top of the turkey, then layer with the tomato and mozzarella slices. Cover with the red onion rings and sprinkle with the arugula leaves. Top with the olives and finish with a layer of the cheese. Place the bread loaf top back on and press down firmly.

- Wrap in wax paper and refrigerate until needed. Cut into wedges to serve.

---

10 Mini Picnic Rolls

Cut 2 crusty rolls in half horizontally. Pull out the soft bread from the bottom of each and fill with 2 slices each of wafer-thin ham and mozzarella cheese, 3 slices of tomato, and 4 slices of cucumber. Lightly spread the top of each with 1 teaspoon mayonnaise, then place the top of the roll back on the bottom. Press down well, cut in half, and secure with a toothpick, if necessary. Serve half a roll per child.

20 Warm Ciabatta Picnic Loaf

Cut 1 ciabatta loaf horizontally about one-third of the way down. Pull out half of the soft bread from the bottom of the loaf. Drain 1 (12 oz) jar of roasted peppers and place in the bottom of the ciabatta in layers with 5 oz drained and sliced mozzarella cheese and 2 oz salami. Place on a baking sheet, put the top back on, and secure with toothpicks. Place in a preheated oven, at 400 °F, for 5–10 minutes to warm through. Serve in chunky slices.

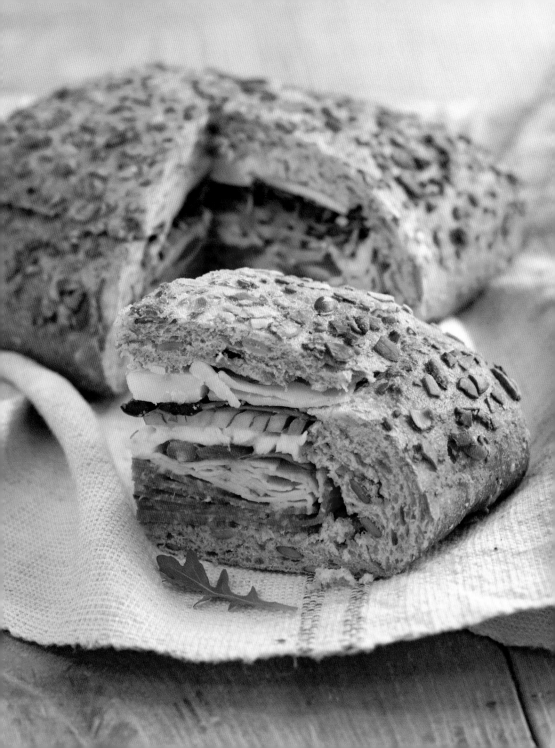

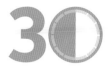

Crunchy Chicken Pesto Dippers

Serves 4

⅔ cup prepared pesto

1 lb boneless, skinless chicken breast, cut into chunks or thick slices

1 cup couscous

3 tablespoons crème fraîche or Greek yogurt

vegetable crudités, such as red bell pepper and carrot sticks, to serve (optional)

- Place 1 tablespoon of the pesto in a small bowl and reserve. Put the remaining pesto in a mixing bowl with the chicken and toss well to coat the chicken.

- Put the couscous in a bowl. Lightly coat the chicken, one piece at a time, in the couscous, then place on a baking sheet, spaced apart. Bake in a preheated oven, at 400°F, for 20–25 minutes, until the chicken is tender and cooked through and the outer coating is golden.

- Meanwhile, mix the crème fraîche or yogurt with the reserved pesto and place in a small bowl on a serving platter with the crudités. Using tongs, transfer the crunchy pesto chicken on to the serving platter. Serve while warm, with decorated toothpicks, for kids to share.

---

1 **Chicken Skewers with Warm Pesto Dip** Heat ⅓ cup olive oil in a skillet and cook ¼ cup pine nuts for 2 minutes, until golden. Place ¼ cup grated Parmesan cheese in a food processor with 1½ cups fresh basil leaves, pour over the hot oil and pine nuts, and process until smooth. Add 3 tablespoons ricotta cheese and process again. Pour into a small heatproof serving dish and serve with freshly cut vegetable crudités and store-bought chicken skewers or cooked chicken nuggets for dipping.

2 **Pesto Chicken Couscous** Place an envelope of flavored couscous in a bowl. Pour over enough hot water to cover, according to the package directions, and set aside to swell for 15 minutes. Meanwhile, cut 1 lb boneless, skinless chicken breasts into chunks and toss with ¼ cup pesto to coat. Place the chunks on an aluminum foil-lined broiler rack and cook under a preheated broiler for 10–12 minutes, turning once, until golden and cooked through. Toss into the couscous along with 2 tablespoons toasted pine nuts and a handful of chopped basil leaves.

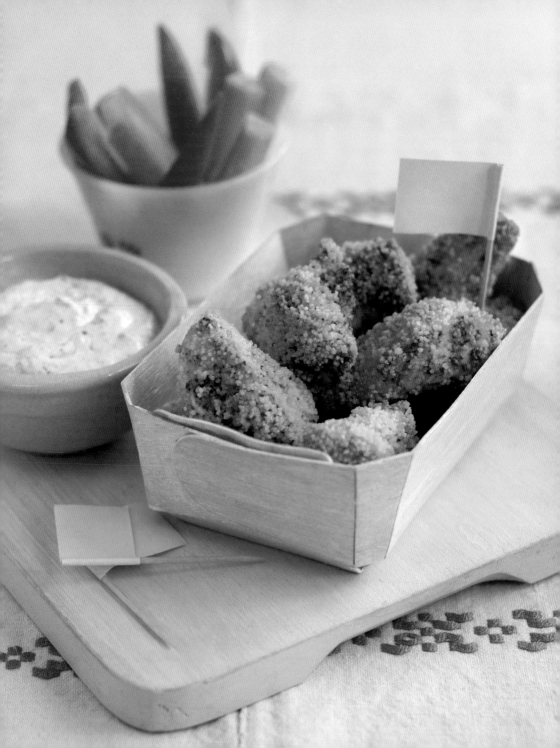

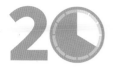

Brown Rice Salad with Peanuts and Raisins

Serves 4

1 cup instant brown rice
bunch of scallions,
  coarsely chopped
1 cup raisins
1 red bell pepper, cored,
  seeded, and sliced
¾ cup roasted peanuts
2 tablespoons dark soy sauce
1 tablespoon sesame oil

- Cook the rice in a saucepan of lightly salted boiling water for 15–18 minutes, until tender.

- Meanwhile, place the scallions, raisins, red bell pepper, and peanuts in a large bowl and toss with the soy sauce and sesame oil until well coated.

- Once the rice is cooked, drain it in a strainer and rinse with cold water until cold. Once cold and drained, add to the other ingredients and toss well to coat and mix.

- Turn into a serving bowl and serve, or place in a lunchbox with slices of cheese or meat to serve alongside, if desired.

 Speedy Raisin and Peanut Rice Salad

Place 1¼ cups fresh cooked rice in a bowl with 1 cup raisins, 2 large, peeled and shredded carrots, and ⅓ cup chopped parsley. Add ½ cup coarsely chopped peanuts and toss well.

 Fruit and Nut Pilaf Rice

Cook 1¼ cups instant brown rice in a large saucepan of lightly salted boiling water for 15–18 minutes, until tender. Meanwhile, heat 3 tablespoons olive oil in a skillet over high heat and cook 1 sliced red onion and 1 small cored, seeded, and sliced red bell pepper for 4–5 minutes, until soft. Add ½ cup pine nuts and 1 bunch of coarsely chopped scallions and cook for another 2–3 minutes, until the pine nuts are golden. Once the rice is cooked, drain well. Add the hot rice to the pan with the bell peppers and pine nuts and toss well. Add 1 cup raisins and ½ cup chopped dried apricots. Toss well, then add ¼ cup chopped parsley and serve hot.

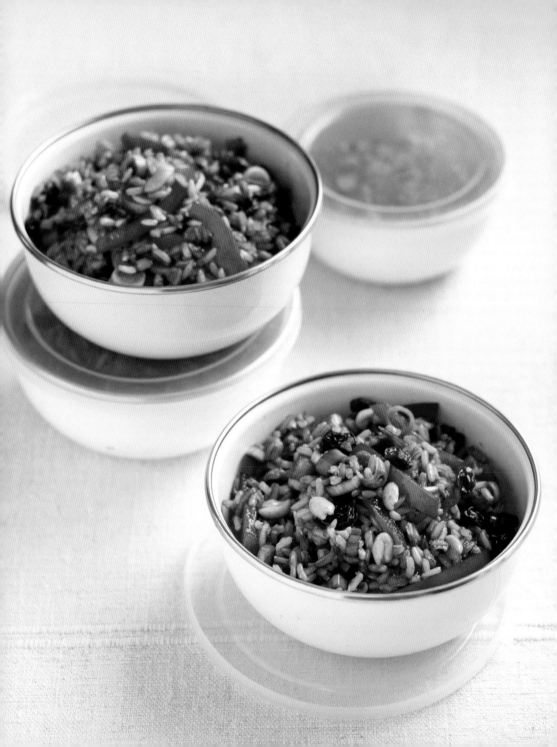

30 Ricotta and Tomato Biscuits

Makes 8

4 cups all-purpose flour, plus
extra for dusting

4 teaspoons baking powder

1 cup ricotta cheese, plus extra
to serve (optional)

1 egg

1 cup milk

3 tablespoons chopped mixed
herbs, such as basil, parsley,
and oregano

4 sun-dried tomatoes, drained
and coarsely chopped

beaten egg, to glaze

1 tablespoon sesame seeds

salt and black pepper

butter, to serve (optional)

- Sift the flour and baking powder into a food processor and season with a little salt and black pepper. Place the ricotta, egg, milk, herbs, and tomatoes in a separate bowl and beat together well. Add the ricotta mixture to the flour and process to form a soft dough. Turn out onto a lightly floured surface and roll out to about 1 inch thick.

- Stamp out 8 biscuits using a 2½ inch cutter and place on a baking sheet. Brush with a little milk and sprinkle with sesame seeds. Bake in a preheated oven, at 400°F, for 15 minutes, until golden and risen.

- Serve warm with butter or extra ricotta for spreading.

---

1 **Quick Ricotta and Tomato-Topped Biscuits** Cut 4 prepared cheese biscuits in half. Mix 1 cup ricotta cheese with 5 coarsely chopped sun-dried tomatoes and ¼ cup chopped basil. Spread spoonfuls of the mixture on each of the biscuit halves, top with 2 pitted ripe black olives, and serve with extra basil leaves to garnish, if desired. The biscuits can be warmed in a preheated oven, at 400°F, for 5 minutes while making the ricotta topping, if preferred.

2 **Biscuit Wedges with Ricotta and Tomato Topping** Make up 1 (8 oz) package biscuit mix according to the package directions, using egg and milk. Roll out into a rough circle and cut into 8 wedges. Place the wedges, spaced well apart, on a baking sheet and brush with milk. Sprinkle with 1 tablespoon sesame seeds and bake in a preheated oven, at 450°F, for 10–12 minutes, until golden. Meanwhile, mix ¾ cup ricotta cheese, 4 coarsely chopped sun-dried tomatoes, and 3 tablespoons basil leaves in a bowl. To serve, cut open the warm biscuits and spread with the herb and tomato ricotta mixture.

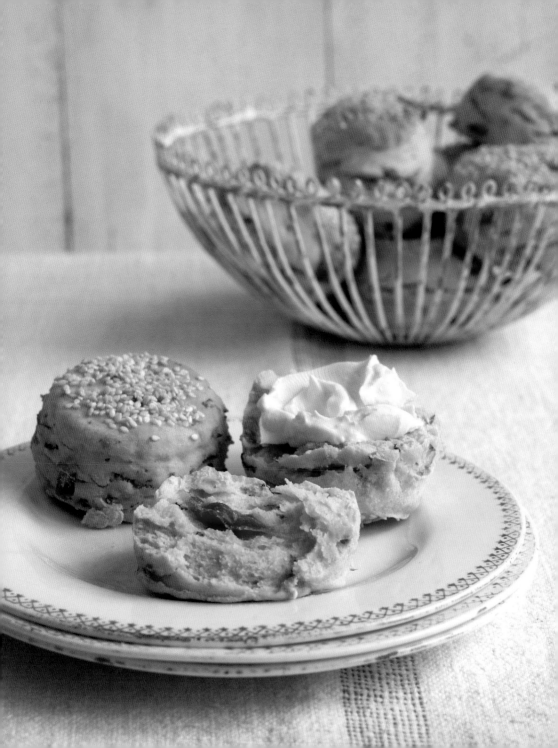

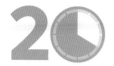

Honeyed Duck Strips in Lettuce "Boats"

Serves 4

2 tablespoons sesame oil

2 (6 oz) duck breasts, cut into thin strips

2 teaspoons Chinese five spice powder

2 tablespoons dark soy sauce

2 tablespoons honey

2 tablespoons toasted sesame seeds

8 butterhead lettuce leaves

To garnish

4 scallions, finely chopped

1 small carrot, peeled and shredded

crusty bread, to serve (optional)

- Heat the oil in a heavy skillet. Toss the duck strips with the Chinese five spice powder in a bowl, then cook over high heat for 8–10 minutes, until cooked and crispy. Add the soy sauce and honey and cook for another 2 minutes to coat in the sticky glaze. Sprinkle with the sesame seeds and keep warm.

- Wash and pat dry the lettuce leaves and place on a serving board. Place spoonfuls of the duck into the leaves, then garnish each with the scallions and carrot.

- Serve with crusty bread, if desired.

Honeyed Duck Stir-Fry

Heat 2 tablespoons sesame oil in a large, heavy skillet and cook 6 oz thinly sliced duck breast over high heat for 4 minutes. Add 1 (1 lb) package prepared stir-fry vegetables to the skillet with 2 teaspoons Chinese five spice powder and stir-fry for 3–4 minutes, until tender but still retaining their shape. Add 1 tablespoon honey, 2 tablespoons sesame seeds, and 2 tablespoons soy sauce and stir-fry for 2 minutes, then serve in warmed bowls.

Honey Duck Pilaf

Cook 1¼ cups instant white or long-grain rice in a large saucepan of lightly salted boiling water according to package directions, until tender. Meanwhile, heat 2 tablespoons sesame oil in a large, heavy skillet and cook 2 (6 oz) duck breasts, thinly sliced, over high heat for 5 minutes, until beginning to turn golden. Add 2 teaspoons Chinese five spice powder and cook for another 3–4 minutes. Add 4 finely shredded scallions and 1 large peeled and finely shredded carrot and cook over high heat for 2 minutes. Add 1 tablespoon dark soy sauce and 2 tablespoons honey, increase the heat, and cook for another 2 minutes. Drain the rice, then add to the duck mixture and stir for 2 minutes. Serve sprinkled with chopped cilantro, if desired.

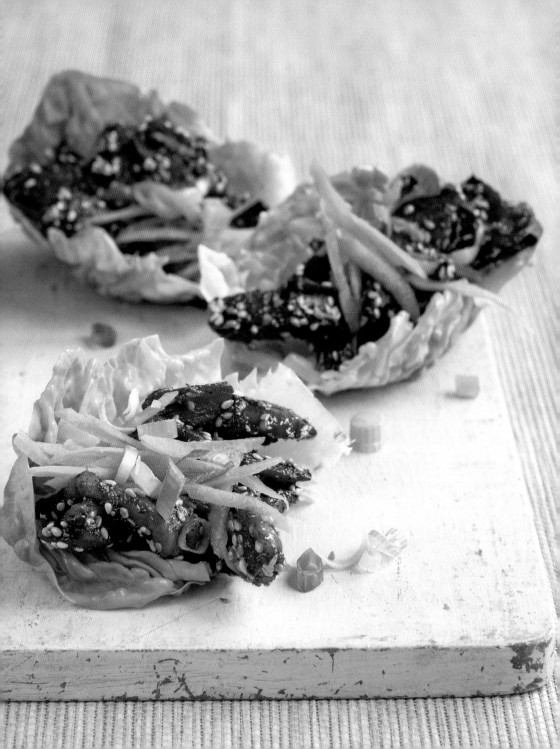

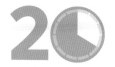

Pineapple and Chunky Ham Skewers

Serves 4

1 lb cured ham

2 tablespoons olive oil

1 teaspoon whole-grain mustard

2 tablespoons honey

1 tablespoon chopped parsley

½ pineapple, peeled, cored, and cut into 16 chunks

vegetable crudités, to serve (optional)

- Cut the ham into 24 chunky pieces. Heat 1 tablespoon of the oil in a heavy skillet and cook the ham over medium-high heat for 5–7 minutes, until cooked through and golden in places. Add the honey and parsley and toss to coat the ham pieces. Keep warm.

- In a separate skillet, heat the remaining oil and cook the pineapple chunks over high heat for 4–5 minutes, until golden and hot.

- Thread 3 chunks of ham and 2 chunks of pineapple onto 8 small bamboo skewers and serve with crudités.

 Warm Ham and Pineapple Pita Breads Lightly toast 4 pita breads and keep warm. Heat 1 stick butter in a skillet and cook 1 (8 oz) can pineapple chunks, drained, over high heat for 5 minutes, until piping hot and golden in places. Add 6 oz chopped ham and cook for another 3 minutes, until beginning to turn golden in places. Mix 2 tablespoons honey with 1 teaspoon whole-grain mustard and toss into the skillet. Load into the pita breads and serve with salad, if desired.

 Pineapple and Ham Stir-Fry Heat 2 tablespoons olive oil in a wok or skillet and cook 12 oz cured ham, cut into 1 inch cubes, for 10 minutes, until golden and cooked through. Add ½ pineapple, peeled and cut into chunks, and stir-fry over high heat for another 5 minutes, until the pineapple is beginning to turn golden. Core, seed, and cut 1 red and 1 green bell pepper into chunks, add to the wok, and stir-fry for 3–4 minutes, until beginning to soften. Mix 1 tablespoon whole-grain mustard with 3 tablespoons honey and 3 tablespoons chopped parsley, pour into the wok, and cook, stirring and tossing, for another 2–3 minutes, until the ham and pineapple are coated in the mustard glaze. Serve with egg noodles.

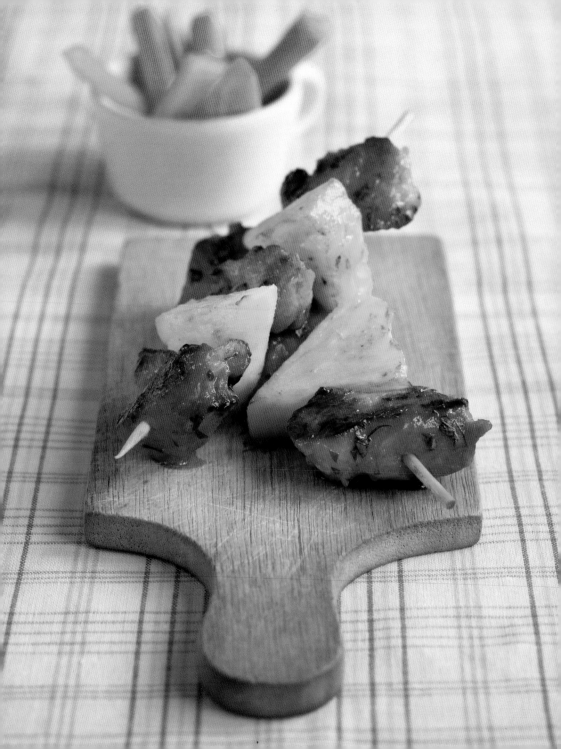

30 Mini Brie and Tomato Quiches

Serves 4

1 sheet rolled dough pie crust

16 cherry tomatoes

6 oz Brie, cut into cubes

1 tablespoon chopped parsley

2 eggs

2 tablespoons crème fraîche
   or sour cream

black pepper

salad or baked beans, to serve
   (optional)

- Unroll the dough and cut into four 5 inch squares. Use to line a 4-cup shallow muffin pan and press down. Put 4 tomatoes in each and divide the Brie among them. Mix together the parsley, eggs, and crème fraîche or sour cream, beating until smooth, and season with a little black pepper. Pour into the pastry shells to just cover the cheese.

- Bake in a preheated oven, at 400°F, for 20 minutes, until golden and puffed, and the pastry is cooked.

- Serve hot with a simple salad or baked beans, if desired.

---

1 Brie and Tomato Crostini

Cut a ciabatta loaf in half both horizontally and lengthwise to make 4 pieces. Drizzle each with 1 tablespoon olive oil and place on a baking sheet. Cook under a preheated hot broiler for 1 minute, until beginning to toast. Remove and top each with 2 oz Brie slices and 6 cherry tomatoes. Season with black pepper. Broil for another 4–5 minutes, until the tomatoes split slightly and the Brie melts and turns golden, then serve.

2 Baked brie and Tomato

Divide 12 cherry tomatoes among 4 ramekins. Cut 6 oz Brie into chunks, then divide among the ramekins. Beat 4 eggs with 1 tablespoon chopped parsley and 2 tablespoons crème fraîche or sour cream and season generously with black pepper. Pour the egg mixture over the tomatoes and Brie in the ramekins, then place on a baking sheet and bake in a preheated oven, at 425°F, for 15 minutes, until well puffed up and turning pale golden. Let cool slightly, then serve on small plates with crusty bread.

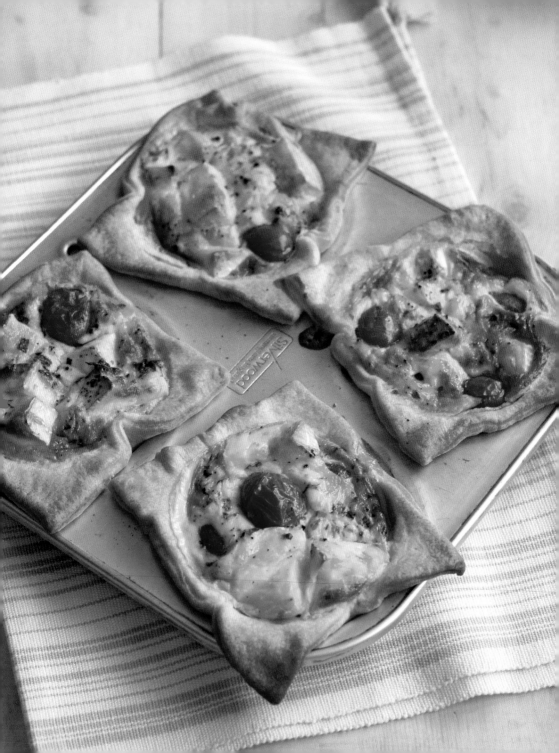

30 Curried Chicken Couscous Salad

Serves 4

1 cup couscous

3 tablespoons olive oil

1 red onion, sliced

12 oz boneless, skinless chicken breast, thinly sliced

bunch of scallions, cut into strips

¼ cup mild curry paste

2 tablespoons water

1 ripe mango, peeled, pitted, and cut into chunks

¼ cup chopped cilantro (optional)

Greek yogurt or plain yogurt, to serve (optional)

- Place the couscous in a bowl and pour over enough lightly salted water to just cover. Set aside for 20 minutes to swell.

- Meanwhile, heat the oil in a skillet and cook the red onion and chicken slices over high heat for 5 minutes, then reduce the heat, add the scallions, and cook for 3–4 minutes, until softened and cooked through. Keep warm.

- In a separate skillet, heat the curry paste over low heat until softened, adding the measured water to loosen. Drain the couscous and transfer to the skillet with the curry paste and toss and stir to coat and heat for about 2 minutes.

- Toss the chicken and onions into the curried couscous with the mango and cilantro, if using, and toss again before serving with spoonfuls of yogurt, if desired.

 Curried Chicken and Mint Couscous

Thinly slice 8 oz boneless, skinless chicken breasts. Heat 3 tablespoons olive oil in a large, heavy skillet and cook the chicken over high heat for 5 minutes, until golden and cooked through. Add 2 tablespoons mild curry paste with 2 tablespoons water and heat for 2 minutes, until hot. Transfer to a mixing bowl. Add 2 cups cooked couscous, 8 halved cherry tomatoes, and ½ cup sliced cucumbers and toss into the chicken with 2 tablespoons chopped mint. Serve with spoonfuls of tzatziki.

 Curried Chicken Salad with Couscous Place ½ (8 oz) package flavored couscous in a bowl. Pour over hot water according to the package directions and set aside to swell. Meanwhile, place ⅓ cup mayonnaise in a bowl with ¼ cup plain yogurt and 3 tablespoons mild curry paste and mix together. Add 12 oz store-bought, cooked chicken, 5 coarsely chopped scallions, 1 small peeled, pitted, and coarsely chopped mango, and ¼ cup chopped cilantro. Stir well to coat in the curried mayonnaise and serve alongside the couscous.

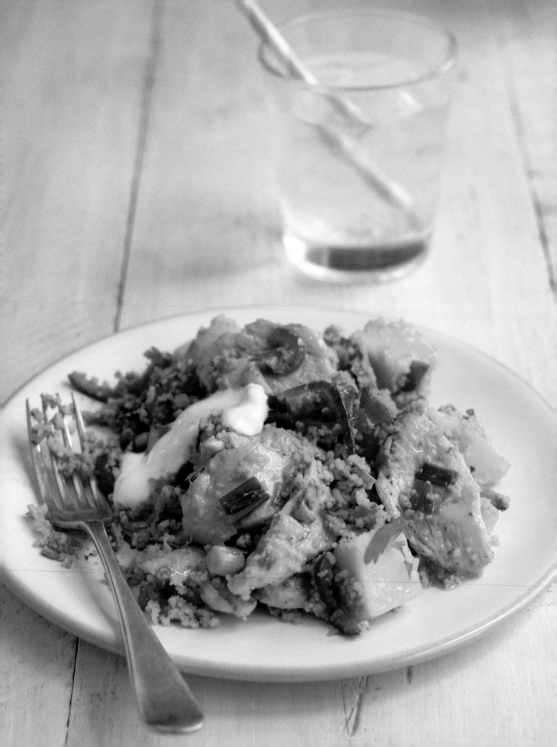

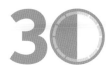

30 Vegetable and Cheese Turnovers

Makes 4

2 sheets store-bought rolled
   dough pie crust
flour, for dusting
2 tablespoons butter, melted
1 (1 lb) frozen prepared mixed
   vegetables for soup, thawed
   and coarsely chopped into
   about ½ inch cubes if too large
1 cup shredded sharp
   cheddar cheese
1 tablespoon dried thyme
beaten egg, to glaze
black pepper

- Roll out the dough on a lightly floured surface and cut out four 10 inch circles, using a plate, if necessary.

- Put the melted butter and oil in a bowl with the vegetables and toss well. Season with plenty of black pepper and toss again. Add the cheese and thyme and toss well. Divide the vegetable and cheese mixture among the 4 circles of dough. Dampen the rims of the pastry, using a brush and a little water, then lift the dough edges up and over the filling to meet one another and pinch together to hold the edges together. Place on a large baking sheet and crimp the edges using your fingers.

- Brush with beaten egg and bake in a preheated oven, at 400°F, for 20 minutes, until golden and cooked through. The vegetables cook in their own steam inside the pastry and should be tender.

1 Cheesy Vegetable Soup Place 1 (1 lb) package frozen prepared soup vegetable mix in a saucepan with 2½ cups vegetable stock and bring to a boil. Cover, reduce the heat, and simmer for 8 minutes, then transfer to a food processor with ¾ cup shredded cheddar cheese, 2 tablespoons thyme leaves, and 1 teaspoon Dijon mustard and process until smooth and thick. Divide between 2 bowls and serve with warm crusty bread.

2 Carrot and Cheese Tarts Unroll 1 sheet store-bought rolled dough pie crust, stamp out four 5 inch circles, and use to line a 4-cup shallow muffin pan. Bake in a preheated oven, at 400°F, for 10 minutes, until pale golden. Meanwhile, sprinkle 2 large peeled and coarsely chopped carrots in a roasting pan and toss with 3 tablespoons olive oil. Roast at the top of the oven above the pastry tart shells for 12 minutes, until lightly charred in places and tender. Meanwhile, cut 4 oz cheddar cheese into small cubes and place in a bowl with 1 tablespoon olive oil and 1 tablespoon chopped thyme. Add the roasted carrots to the bowl and toss to warm and slightly melt the cheese. Divide the filling among the tarts and serve warm.

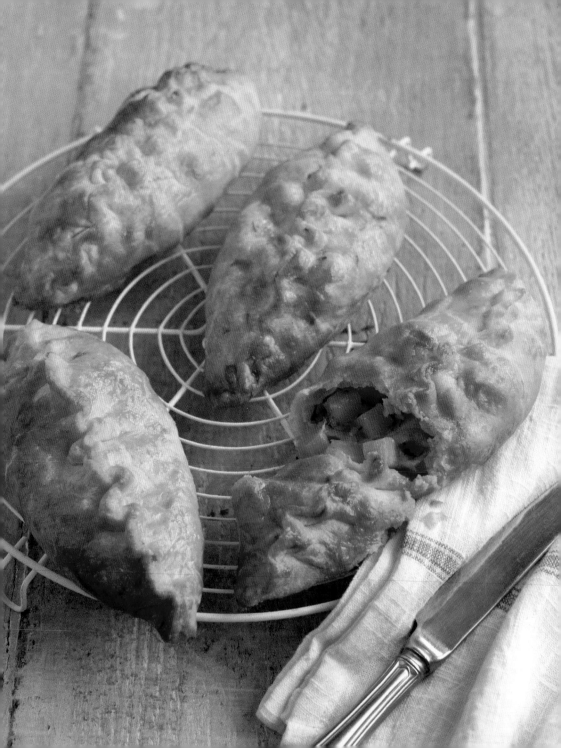

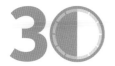

30 Sticky Chicken Drumsticks with Homemade Coleslaw

Serves 4

2 tablespoons honey

1 tablespoon whole-grain mustard

3 tablespoons ketchup

2 teaspoons dark soy sauce

1 tablespoon olive oil

8 chicken drumsticks

For the coleslaw

¼ small savoy cabbage, shredded

2 large carrots, peeled and shredded

2 tablespoons chopped parsley

⅓ cup mayonnaise

¼ cup crème fraîche, sour cream, or plain yogurt

1 tablespoon water

black pepper

bread rolls, to serve (optional)

- Place the honey, mustard seeds, ketchup, soy sauce, and oil in a large mixing bowl and blend well. Add the chicken drumsticks and toss in the marinade. Place in a roasting pan, brush over any remaining marinade, and cook in a preheated oven, at 425°F, for 20–25 minutes, until golden and cooked through.

- Meanwhile, make the coleslaw. Place the shredded cabbage, carrots, and parsley in a mixing bowl and toss together. Mix together the mayonnaise, crème fraîche or alternative choice, and measured water in a separate bowl, then season well with black pepper. Spoon the dressing over the coleslaw, then mix and toss well to coat.

- Serve the chicken drumsticks with the coleslaw and bread rolls, if desired.

---

1 Chicken Coleslaw Pita Breads

Shred ¼ green or savoy cabbage and place in a bowl with 2 peeled and shredded carrots. Toss in 2 tablespoons chopped parsley. Tear 8 oz store-bought cooked chicken into shreds and add to the coleslaw mix. Add 3 tablespoons raisins. Mix ⅓ cup mayonnaise with 2 tablespoons water, stir into the chicken coleslaw, and mix to coat. Pile into warm toasted pita breads and serve.

2 Sticky Chicken Skewers with Red Coleslaw

If using wooden skewers, first presoak for 30 minutes. Slice 8 oz boneless, skinless chicken breast into long, thin slices. Place 2 tablespoons honey, 1 tablespoon whole-grain mustard, 3 tablespoons ketchup, 2 teaspoons dark soy sauce, and 1 tablespoon olive oil in a bowl and mix well. Add the chicken strips and toss well. Thread onto 4 metal or presoaked wooden skewers, then cook under a preheated medium broiler for 10 minutes, turning occasionally, until golden and cooked through. Meanwhile, to make the red coleslaw, place ¼ small shredded red cabbage in a bowl with 1 large peeled and shredded carrot and ⅓ cup mayonnaise mixed with 3 tablespoons water. Toss well to coat in the dressing. Serve the skewers with the coleslaw and bread rolls, if desired.

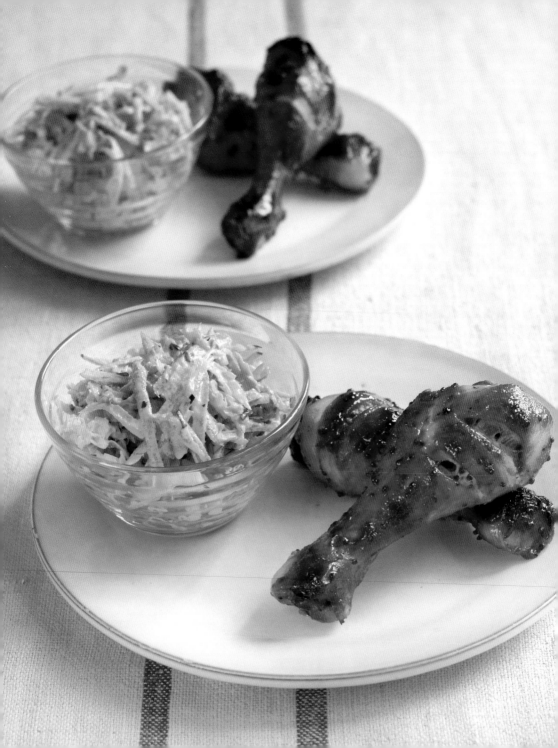

30 Mini Falafel Burgers

Serves 4

2 tablespoons sunflower oil
1 small onion, finely chopped
1 garlic clove, crushed
1 (15 oz) can chickpeas,
  rinsed and drained
1 teaspoon ground cumin
1 teaspoon ground coriander
3 tablespoons chopped cilantro
1 egg yolk
¼ cup Greek yogurt or
  plain yogurt
1 teaspoon mint sauce
salt and black pepper

To serve

8 warm toasted mini pita breads
lettuce leaves
8 cherry tomatoes, halved

- Heat 1 tablespoon of the oil in a large skillet. Add the onion and cook over low heat for 5 minutes, until softened. Transfer to a large mixing bowl with the chickpeas and ground spices and mash, using a fork or potato masher, until the chickpeas are broken down. Stir in the chopped cilantro and season to taste. Add the egg yolk, then squash the mixture together with your hands.

- Mold the mixture into 8 small balls, then flatten into patty shapes. Heat the remaining oil in a skillet and cook the falafels for 3 minutes on each side, until golden brown and firm to the touch.

- Mix the yogurt with the mint sauce and spoon it over the falafels (hot or cold). Serve with the mini pita breads, lettuce leaves, and tomatoes.

---

1 Quick Chickpea and Spinach Stir-Fry

Heat 2 tablespoons oil in a saucepan and cook 1 chopped onion for 2 minutes. Add 1 (15 oz) can chickpeas, rinsed and drained, and 1 (12 oz) package baby spinach leaves and cook for 2 minutes. Add ½ teaspoon ground cumin, ½ teaspoon ground coriander, and ½ teaspoon minced garlic and cook for 2 minutes. Add 8 halved cherry tomatoes and cook for 1 minute. Pour in 1¾ cups coconut milk, heat for 2 minutes, and serve with warm pita bread.

2 Chickpea and Cilantro Dahl

Heat 2 tablespoons sunflower oil in a large skillet and cook 1 small finely chopped onion and 1 crushed garlic clove for 3–4 minutes, until softened. Add 1 (15 oz) can chickpeas, rinsed and drained, 1 teaspoon ground cumin, 1 teaspoon ground coriander, and 3 tablespoons chopped cilantro and cook for 2 minutes. Add 2½ cups vegetable stock, bring to a boil, and cook for 5 minutes. Transfer to a food processor and process until smooth. Make a raita by mixing ¼ cup plain yogurt with 1 teaspoon mint sauce and spoon it over the dahl. Serve with warm naan or pita breads cut into fingers for the kids to dip.

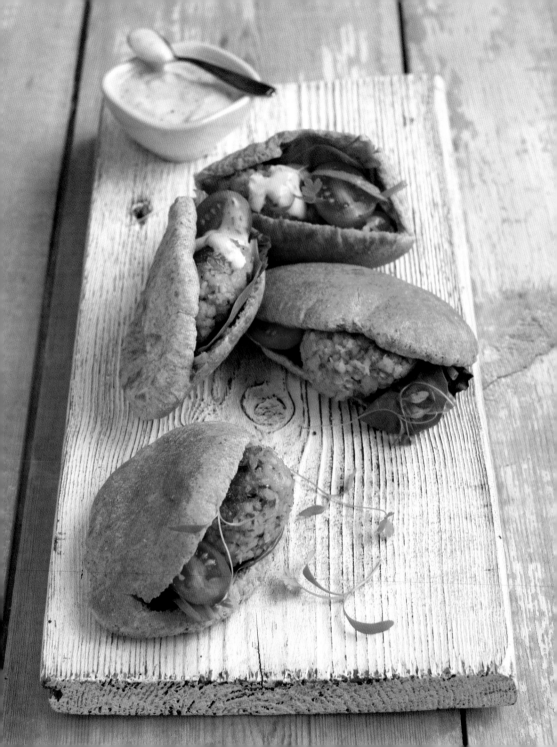

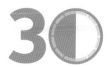

30 Pinwheels with Cream Cheese Dip

Makes 24

1 sheet ready-to-bake
  puff pastry
2 tablespoons yeast extract,
  or Worcestershire sauce,
  for sprinkling
2 tablespoons chopped parsley,
  to garnish

For the cream cheese dip

1 cup cream cheese
⅓ cup milk
2 tablespoons chopped chives
1 tablespoon whole-grain mustard
black pepper

- Unroll the pastry on a large cutting board. Spread thinly with the yeast extract, or sprinkle with Wocestersire sauce, right to the edges, then roll up tightly along its width. Using a sharp knife, cut the pastry into 24 slices and place well apart on a baking sheet. Bake in a preheated oven, at 425°F, for 15–18 minutes, until golden and puffed.

- Meanwhile, make the cream cheese dip. Place the cream cheese in a bowl with the milk and chives. Season generously with black pepper, add the mustard, and mash well. Place in a small bowl and serve alongside the warm pinwheels.

---

1 **Grilled Cheese Sandwiches** Spread one side of 2 slices of bread with a little butter, then sprinkle with Worcestershire sauce, if desired. Layer the other piece of bread with a slice of cheddar, Swiss, or American cheese and top with the buttered slice, face down. Heat 1 tablespoon butter in a large skillet and cook the sandwich over high heat for 1 minute, until golden, then turn it over and cook for 1 minute. Remove from the skillet and cut into triangles to serve. Repeat to make 4 sandwiches.

2 **Cheese and Parsley Open Tarts** Unroll 1 sheet ready-to-bake puff pastry, cut into 4 equal rectangles, and place on a baking sheet. Bake in a preheated oven, at 425°F, for 10–12 minutes, until golden and puffed. Meanwhile, grate 6 oz cheddar cheese and toss with 1 tablespoon chopped parsley. Remove the pastry from the oven, press down the centers, and sprinkle each with a little Worchestershire sauce, if desired. Sprinkle with the cheese mixture and parsley and return to the oven for 5 minutes, until melted. Serve with cherry tomatoes, if desired.

KID-BREA-KUR

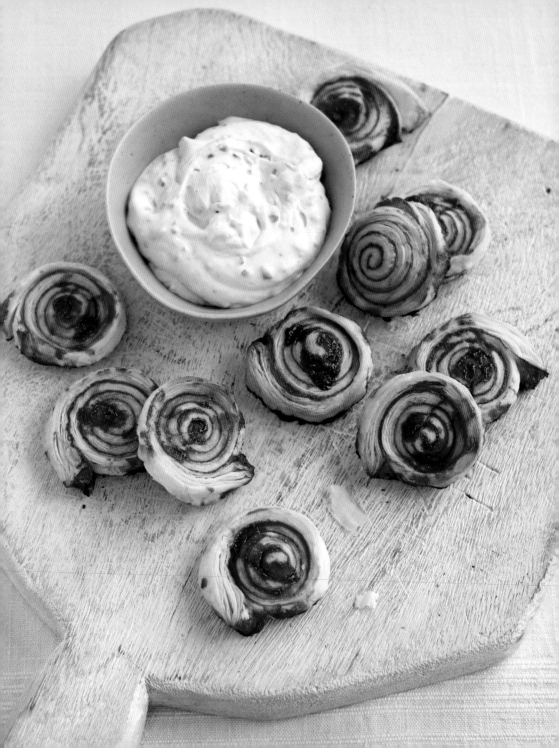

30 Pepperoni and Bell Pepper Rolls

Makes 8

10 oz of pizza crust mix
2 tablespoons chopped oregano
flour, for dusting
1 tablespoon olive oil
¼ small red bell pepper, cored,
  seeded, and sliced
¼ small yellow bell pepper, cored,
  seeded, and sliced
¼ small green bell pepper, cored,
  seeded and sliced
2 oz pepperoni, coarsely chopped
¼ cup shredded cheddar cheese
  or mozzarella cheese

- Place the pizza crust mix in a bowl with the oregano, add warm water according to the package directions, and mix to form a smooth dough. Turn out onto a lightly floured surface and knead until smooth.

- Heat the oil in a heavy skillet and cook the bell peppers over medium heat for 4–5 minutes, until soft, then add the pepperoni and cook for another minute.

- Divide the dough into 8 pieces and make a well in the center of each. Divide the bell peppers and pepperoni among the dough pieces and coarsely knead through the dough. Shape each into a rough ball and place on a baking sheet.

- Sprinkle with the cheddar or mozzarella and bake in a preheated oven, at 425°F, for 20 minutes, until golden and cooked through; the crust should sound hollow when tapped. Serve warm.

---

10 Broiled Pepperoni Pizza-Style Rolls

Cut 2 ciabatta rolls in half and place on an auluminum foil-lined broiler rack, cut side up. Cook under a preheated medium broiler for 1 minute, until the tops are golden and crisp. Top each with 1 piece drained and sliced roasted pepper, 2 slices of pepperoni, and a slice of mozzarella cheese. Broil for 3–4 minutes, until melted and golden, and serve hot.

20 Pepperoni and Roasted Pepper

Pizzas Make up 10 oz of pizza crust mix according to the package directions and divide the dough into 4 pieces. Roll out each piece to a rough circle, about ½ inch thick, and place well apart on 1–2 baking sheets. Drain 1 (12 oz) jar of roasted peppers in oil, then toss in a bowl with ½ teaspoon dried oregano and divide among the pizzas. Top each with 3 slices of pepperoni and 1 tablespoon shredded mozzarella or cheddar cheese. Bake in a preheated oven, at 425°F, for 10 minutes, until golden, and serve hot.

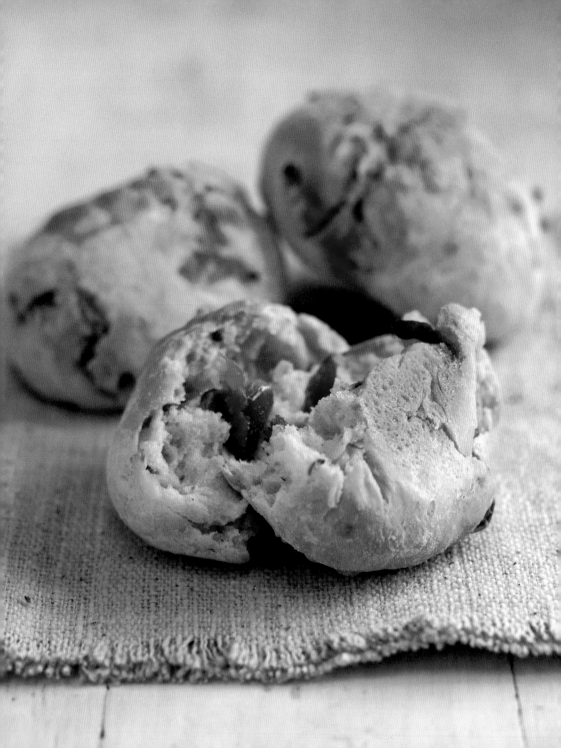

QuickCook

Kids'
Favorites

Recipes listed by cooking time

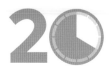 # Pork and Apple Balls

Serves 4

1 small Pippin apple, cored, and
  grated (with skin on)
1 small onion, grated
8 oz ground pork
½ cup whole-wheat
  bread crumbs
3 tablespoons vegetable oil

To serve

tomato chutney
cherry tomato halves

- Place the apple and onion in a bowl with the pork and, using a fork, mash all the ingredients together well. Shape into 16 rough balls. Place the bread crumbs on a plate and roll the balls in the bread crumbs to lightly coat.

- Heat the oil in a large, heavy skillet and cook the balls over medium-high heat for 8–10 minutes, turning frequently, until cooked through. Drain on paper towels.

- Serve warm with tomato chutney and cherry tomatoes, and provide bamboo skewers for dipping the balls in the chutney.

 ### Pork Burgers with Applesauce

Put 12 oz ground pork in a bowl and mix with 1 tablespoon whole-grain mustard and 2 tablespoons chopped parsley. Shape into 4 small, thin patties. Heat 2 tablespoons oil in a skillet and cook the burgers for 2–3 minutes on each side, until golden and cooked through. Use to fill 4 whole-wheat burger buns. Top with applesauce and a small handful of lettuce leaves, if desired.

 ### Pork and Apple Gratins

Heat 1 tablespoon olive oil in a saucepan and cook 8 oz ground pork and 1 small chopped onion over high heat for 5 minutes, until beginning to turn golden. Add 1 small cored and chopped Pippin apple (with skin on) and cook for another 2–3 minutes, stirring continuously to help break up the pork. Add 1¼ cups chicken stock and 1 tablespoon Dijon mustard, stir into the pork, and bring to a boil. Reduce the heat and simmer for 10 minutes. Remove from the heat and divide among 4 shallow ovenproof dishes. Stir in 2 tablespoons butter to 1 cup chilled prepared mashed potato and and season generously with black pepper. Spoon the potato over the pork and apple filling and sprinkle each with 1 teaspoon grated Parmesan cheese. Cook under a preheated hot broiler for 5–10 minutes, until the top is golden and hot. Serve with peas or any green vegetable.

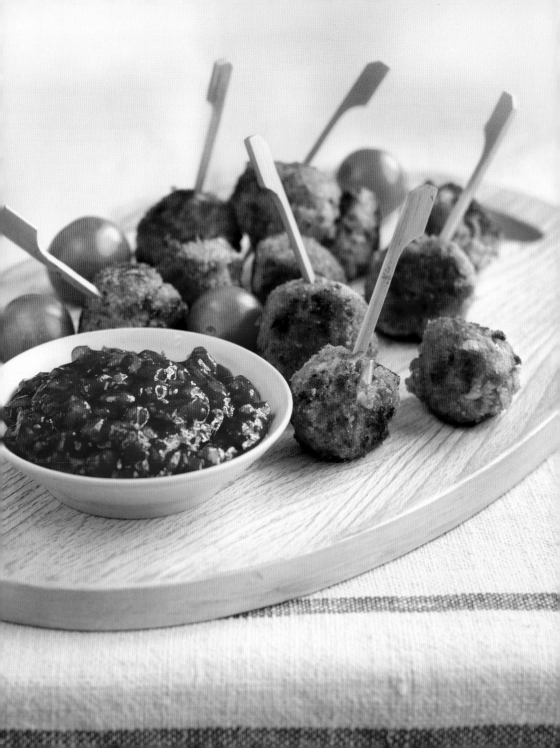

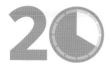 # Chicken and Corn Soup

Serves 4

1 tablespoon sunflower oil
1 boneless, skinless chicken breast
1 onion, chopped
2 cups chicken stock
⅔ cup milk
1 large potato, cut into chunks
1 (11 oz) canned corn kernels, drained
salt and black pepper
crispy bacon pieces, to garnish

- Heat the oil in a saucepan, add the whole chicken breast and the onion, and sauté over low heat for about 5 minutes to soften but not brown. Add the stock, milk, potato, and corn kernels and bring to a boil. Reduce the heat, cover, and simmer for 10 minutes, until the potato and chicken are cooked through.

- Remove the chicken from the pan, place on a board, and shred or chop. Blend the soup with a handheld immersion blender or in a food processor until almost smooth. Season with salt and black pepper, return the chicken to the pan, and reheat.

- Serve sprinkled with crispy bacon pieces.

 Chunky Chicken, Corn, and Bacon Soup Dry-fry 3 chopped bacon slices in a large saucepan. Stir in 2½ cups prepared creamy mushroom soup, 8 oz cooked shredded chicken, and 1 (8¾ oz) can corn kernels, drained. Simmer for 2 minutes, adding a little water if the soup is too thick.

 Creamy Chicken, Corn, and Bacon Casserole Heat 2 tablespoons olive oil in a large skillet and sauté 4 boneless, skinless chicken breasts for 5 minutes, turning once. Remove from the skillet and set aside. Add 1 chopped onion to the skillet with 3 chopped bacon slices and 1 peeled and sliced carrot and sauté for another 5 minutes. Stir in 1 cup crème fraîche or single cream and crumble in a chicken bouillon cube. Heat, stirring, adding a little water, if necessary, to make a smooth sauce. Add 1 (8¾ oz) can corn kernels, drained. Return the chicken to the skillet, cover, and simmer for 10 minutes, until the chicken and vegetables are cooked through. Serve with mashed potatoes.

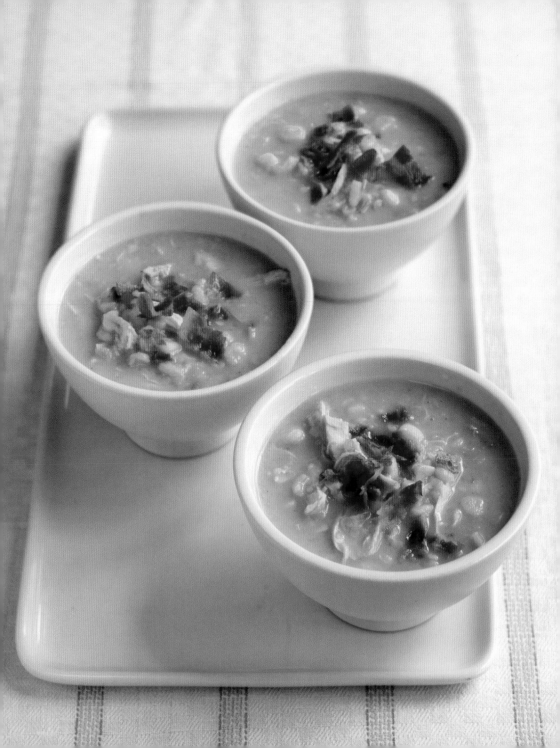

30 Corned Beef and Tomato Pies

Makes 4

1 tablespoon olive oil
1 small onion, finely chopped
1 (12 oz) can corned beef
1 teaspoon Dijon mustard
8 cherry tomatoes, halved
2 tablespoons chopped parsley
1 sheet ready-to-bake
   puff pastry
beaten egg, to glaze

- Heat the oil in a large, heavy skillet and cook the onion for 3–4 minutes, until softened.

- Meanwhile, place the corned beef in a bowl, break it into chunks, using a fork, and mix with the mustard. Add to the skillet with the onion and cook, gently stirring, for 2–3 minutes, until warm, adding the cherry tomato halves for the last minute. Sprinkle with the parsley and gently toss.

- Cut the pastry into four 5 inch squares and four 4 inch squares (rolling the pastry a little wider first, if necessary. Use the larger pieces to line a 4-cup shallow muffin pan with the corners overlapping the cup edges.

- Divide the corned beef-and-tomato mixture among the pastry shells. Lightly brush the edges of each pie with water and place the smaller squares on top as lids. Press down well to adhere, and make a hole in the center of each. Brush with beaten egg and bake in a preheated oven, at 400°F, for 20 minutes, until golden and puffed. Serve.

---

10 Corned Beef and Tomato Hash Pie

Heat 1 tablespoon oil in a skillet. Add 1 (12 oz) can corned beef, mashed, and cook for 2–3 minutes, until softened and hot. Add 10 halved cherry tomatoes and 2 teaspoons Dijon mustard and stir. Place in a shallow gratin dish. Spoon 1 cup prepared mashed potatoes on top of the corned beef. Sprinkle with ½ cup shredded cheddar cheese. Cook under a preheated hot broiler for 2 minutes. Serve with vegetables.

20 Corned Beef and Tomato Tarts

Unroll 1 sheet ready-to-bake puff pastry, cut into 4 equal rectangles, and place on a baking sheet. Lightly score each rectangle ½ inch in from the edge all the way around to produce an inner rectangle (don't cut all the way through). Bake in a preheated oven, at 400°F, for 10–12 minutes, until golden and puffed. Meanwhile, heat 1 tablespoon olive oil in a skillet and cook 1 small finely chopped onion for 3 minutes, then roughly mash 1 (12 oz) can corned beef with 1 teaspoon Dijon mustard, add to the shillet, and cook for 4–5 minutes, until the corned beef is softened and hot. Stir in 8 halved cherry tomatoes for the final 2 minutes. Add 2 tablespoons chopped parsley. Once the tart shells are cooked, remove from the oven. Remove the inner rectangle of pastry and set aside. Divide the corned beef mixture among the tarts and top with the inner pastry rectangles as lids.

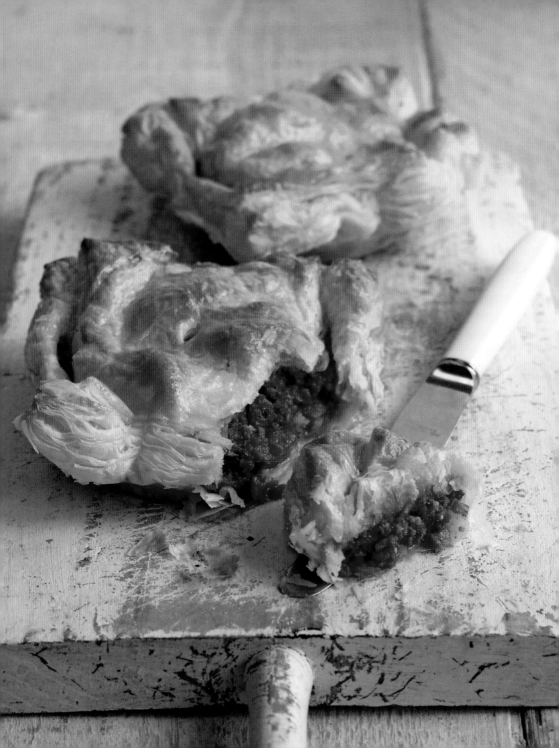

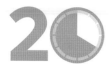 # Tuna and Corn Nuggets

Serves 4

⅔ cup all-purpose flour,
   plus extra for coating
1 extra-large egg
2 tablespoons milk
pinch of chili powder (optional)
1 (5 oz) can chunk-light tuna in
   water, drained and flaked
1 cup drained canned corn kernels
2 scallions, chopped
3 tablespoons sunflower oil
salt and black pepper
ketchup, to serve

- Place the flour in a bowl and make a well in the center. Add the egg, milk, and chili powder, if using, and season with salt and black pepper. Stir well to make a stiff batter.

- Add the tuna, corn, and scallions and stir until evenly mixed. Take tablespoons of the batter, dip them in flour, and roughly shape into 16 nuggets.

- Heat the oil in a large skillet, add the nuggets, and cook, in 2 batches, for about 5 minutes, turning occasionally, until golden. Drain on paper towels and serve with ketchup.

 ### Tuna and Corn Omelet

Heat 2 tablespoons butter in a nonstick skillet. Add 2 chopped scallions and cook for 2 minutes. Beat together 4 eggs, 1 (5 oz) can chunk-light tuna in water, drained and flaked, and 1 (8¾ oz) can corn kernels, drained. Season and pour into the skillet. Dot with 4 halved cherry tomatoes and cook until the egg has set underneath, gently pulling the cooked edges toward the center. When almost set, place the pan under a preheated hot broiler (keeping the handle away from the heat) and cook for 2 minutes. Cut into wedges and serve with crusty bread.

 ### Cheesy Tuna and Corn Baked

Potatoes Scrub 4 small baking potatoes and prick all over with a fork. Cook in the microwave on full power for about 15 minutes, until soft. Cut in half and scoop the potato flesh into a bowl. Coarsely mash the potato flesh with ½ cup shredded cheddar cheese and season with salt and black pepper. Stir in 2 chopped scallions, 1 (5 oz) can tuna, drained and flaked, and 1 (8¾ oz) can corn kernels, drained. Spoon the mixture back into the potato skins, place on an aluminum foil-lined broiler pan, and sprinkle extra cheese on the top. Cook under a preheated medium broiler for about 5 minutes, until the cheese is melted and bubbling. Serve with peas and chopped tomatoes.

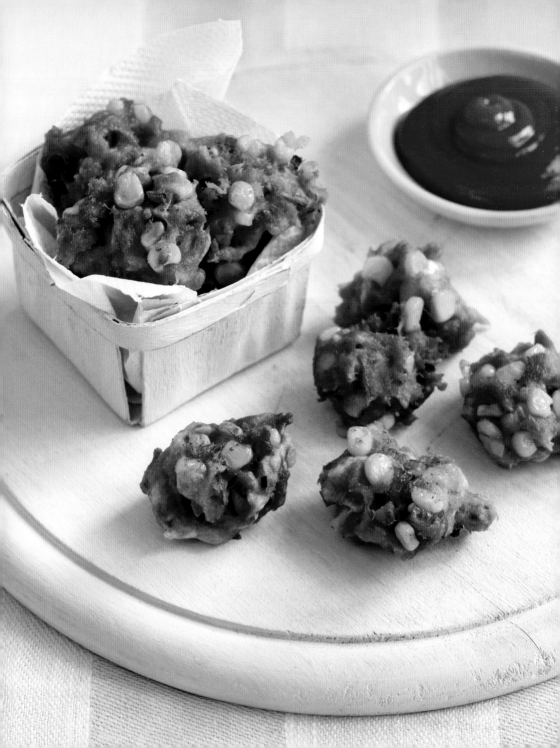

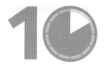 # Sweet Chili and Ginger Shrimp Vegetable Stir-Fry

Serves 4

2 (8 oz) packages instant rice

1 tablespoon sunflower oil

6 scallions, each cut into 3 pieces diagonally and halved lengthwise

1 teaspoon ginger paste

2 cups sugarsnap peas

1 cup frozen soybeans (edamame)

1 head bok choy, leaves separated and shredded

12 oz peeled shrimp

2 tablespoons sweet chili sauce

2 tablespoons soy sauce

- Prepare the rice either by boiling or microwaving, according to the package directions. Meanwhile, heat the oil in a wok or large skillet. Add the scallions, ginger, sugarsnap peas, and soybeans and stir-fry over high heat for 2 minutes.

- Add the bok choy and stir-fry for 1 minute, then add the shrimp and cook for another minute. Mix together the sweet chili sauce and soy sauce, pour into the wok, and heat through. Serve with the rice.

Sweet Chili and Ginger Shrimp Noodles Soak 8 oz rice noodles in boiling water for 2 minutes to soften, then drain. Heat 1 tablespoon sunflower oil in a wok or large skillet, add 6 chopped scallions, 2 cups sugarsnap peas, 1 shredded carrot, 1 cup frozen soybeans (edmame), and 1 head bok choy, leaves separated, and stir-fry for 2 minutes. Add 12 oz cooked, peeled shrimp and stir-fry for 2 minutes. Add ¾ cup coconut milk, 2 tablespoons sweet chili sauce, 2 tablespoons soy sauce, and 1 teaspoon ginger paste, bring to a boil, and simmer gently for 5 minutes. Add the noodles, stir through, and heat for 2 minutes.

Sweet Chili and Ginger Shrimp Skewers with Fried Rice Mix together 2 tablespoons sweet chili sauce, 2 tablespoons soy sauce, 1 teaspoon ginger paste, and the juice of ½ lime. Add 12 oz large, peeled shrimp and stir to coat in the mixture, then let marinate for 10 minutes. Meanwhile, cook 1 cup long-grain rice in a saucepan of lightly salted boiling water according to the package directions, until tender, then drain. Heat 1 tablespoon sunflower oil in a wok or large skillet, add 6 chopped scallions, 2 cups sugarsnap peas, 1 shredded carrot, 1 cup frozen soybeans (edmame), and 1 head of bok choy, leaves separated, and stir-fry over high heat for 2 minutes, until the bok choy has started to wilt. Stir in the drained rice and 2 tablespoons soy sauce and heat through for 2 minutes. Thread the shrimp onto skewers and cook under a preheated medium broiler for 5 minutes, turning occasionally until pink and hot. Serve with the stir-fried rice.

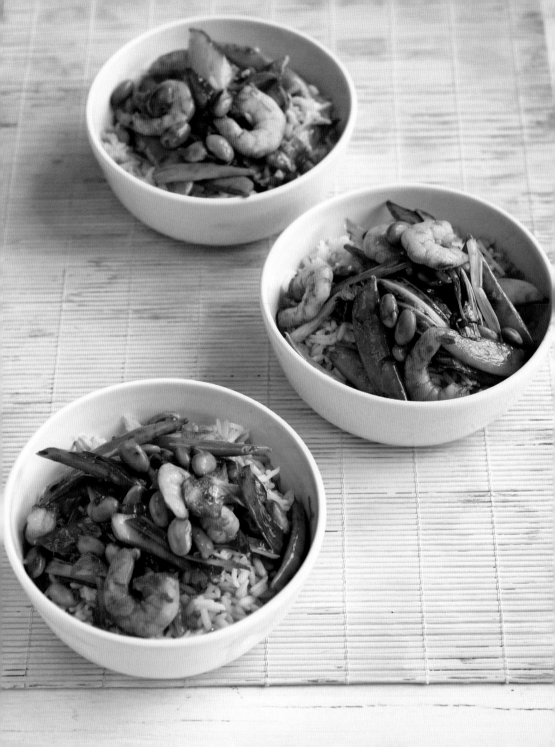

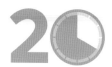

Parmesan Chicken Salad

Serves 4

1½ cups dry white bread crumbs
½ cup grated Parmesan cheese
2 tablespoons all-purpose flour
1 egg, beaten
4 boneless, skinless chicken
breasts, cut in half horizontally
3 tablespoons olive oil
½ romaine lettuce, chopped
¼ cucumber, chopped
1 cup shredded sugarsnap peas
8 cherry tomatoes, halved
¼ cup prepared Caesar salad
dressing
salt and black pepper

- Mix together the bread crumbs and Parmesan on a plate and season with salt and black pepper. Place the flour on another plate and the beaten egg on a third.

- Dip each piece of chicken into the flour, shaking off any excess, then coat in the beaten egg and finally in the bread crumbs, pressing firmly to coat.

- Heat the oil in a large skillet and cook the chicken in batches for 3–4 minutes on each side or until golden, crisp, and cooked through.

- Meanwhile, mix together the lettuce, cucumber, sugarsnap peas, and tomatoes in a salad bowl, then add the Caesar dressing and toss to lightly coat. Serve with the hot chicken.

Chicken and Parmesan Ciabattas

Cut 2 boneless, skinless chicken breasts in half horizontally and season. Heat 2 tablespoons olive oil in a skillet and cook the chicken for about 5 minutes, turning once, until golden and cooked through. Toast 8 slices of ciabatta on both sides. Top 4 slices with shredded crisp lettuce, a drizzle of prepared Caesar salad dressing, and the hot chicken. Add 2 slices of tomato to each and sprinkle with Parmesan cheese shavings. Cover with the remaining bread.

Baked Parmesan Chicken with

Roasted Veg Cut 2 parsnips and 2 carrots into quarters lengthwise. Place on a baking sheet with 8 oz halved new potatoes. Drizzle with 2 tablespoons olive oil and season with salt and black pepper. Roast in a preheated oven, at 425°F, for 25 minutes, turning occasionally, until tender. Meanwhile, cut 3 boneless, skinless chicken breasts into chunky strips. Dip the chicken in beaten egg, then coat in a mixture of ¼ cup uncooked

couscous and ¼ cup grated Parmesan cheese. Spread the chicken out in a single layer on a nonstick baking sheet and cook in the oven with the vegetables for 20 minutes. Serve the chicken and roasted vegetables with green beans or broccoli.

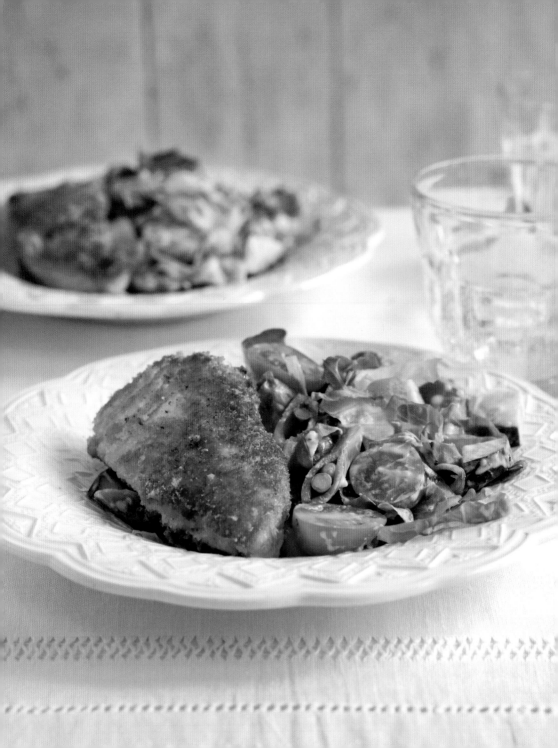

10 Creamy Tomato Soup with Baked Tortilla Chips

Serves 4

2 flour tortillas, cut into triangles
1 tablespoon oil
2 (14½ oz) cans diced tomatoes
2 tablespoons crème fraîche
   or single cream
1¼ cup vegetable stock
2 tablespoons tomato paste
2 tablespoons Worcestershire
   sauce
2 tablespoons thyme
salt and black pepper

- Place the tortilla triangles on a baking sheet and roughly brush with the oil. Season and place in a preheated oven, at 400°F, for 8 minutes.

- Meanwhile, place all the remaining ingredients in a saucepan and bring to a boil. Reduce the heat and simmer for 3–4 minutes, then transfer to a food processor and process until smooth.

- Serve the soup in mugs with the warm baked tortillas to the side.

 Broiled Creamy Tomato Tortillas

Heat 1 tablespoon oil in a saucepan and cook 1 coarsely chopped onion for 3 minutes. Add 1 (14½ oz) can diced tomatoes, 2 tablespoons tomato paste, 2 tablespoons Worcestershire sauce, and 2 tablespoons thyme and bring to a boil, then remove from the heat. Place 1 tortilla on a board and spoon in one-quarter of the tomato mixture. Fold the tortilla into 4, enclosing the filling, and place in a shallow gratin dish. Repeat with 3 more. Season 1 cup crème fraîche or sour cream with black pepper and place spoonfuls over the tortillas. Sprinkle with ¾ cup shredded cheddar cheese and broil for 5–8 minutes.

 Creamy Tomato Stew with Dumplings Heat 1 tablespoon olive oil in a large saucepan (with a tight-fitting lid) and cook 1 large chopped onion for 3–4 minutes. Add 3½ cups (1 lb) whole cherry tomatoes and cook for 2 minutes. Add 2 tablespoons tomato paste, 2 tablespoons Worcestershire sauce, 2 tablespoons thyme, and 2½ cups vegetable stock and bring to a boil. Reduce the heat, cover, and simmer for 5 minutes. Meanwhile, make up ½ (9 oz) package dumpling mix according to the package directions, adding ½ teaspoon dried thyme to the dry mixture. Blend 3 tablespoons cornstarch with ¼ cup water, add to the tomatoes, and stir well to thicken. Add small teaspoons of the dumpling mixture to the pan, cover tightly, and simmer for 15 minutes, until the dumplings are cooked through. Serve the tomato stew and dumplings with spoonfuls of crème fraîche or sour cream.

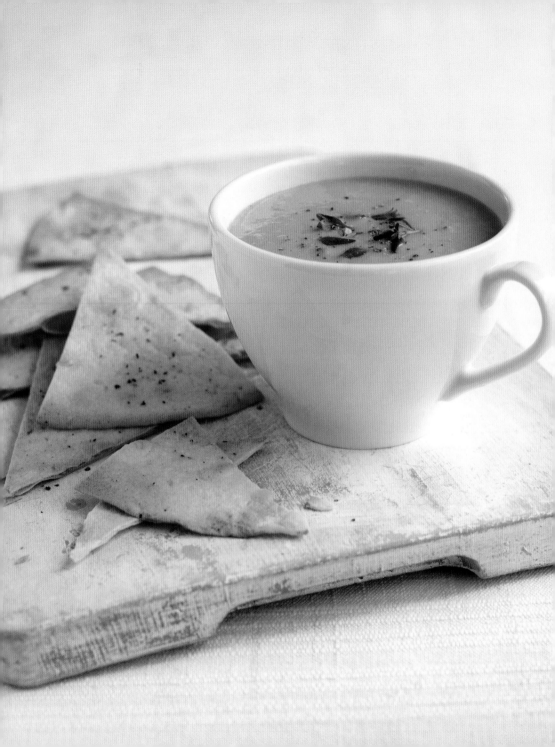

30 Mexican Chicken and Avocado Burgers with Salsa

Serves 4

1 lb boneless, skinless chicken
  breast, coarsely chopped
1 teaspoon dried oregano
1 teaspoon ground cumin
1 teaspoon paprika
½ teaspoon dried
  red pepper flakes
1 tablespoon sunflower oil
4 burger buns
1 avocado, sliced
salt and black pepper

For the salsa

2 ripe tomatoes, chopped
½ small red onion, chopped
small bunch of cilantro, chopped
juice of 1 lime

- Place the chicken in a food processor with the oregano, cumin, paprika, and red pepper flakes. Season with salt and black pepper and process until finely chopped. Shape the mixture into 4 patties and set aside.

- To make the salsa, mix together the tomatoes, red onion, cilantro, and lime juice and season with salt and black pepper.

- Heat the oil in a large skillet, add the chicken burgers, and cook for 5–8 minutes on each side, until golden and cooked through.

- Halve and toast the cut sides of the burger buns. Serve the burgers in the buns topped with slices of avocado and a spoonful of salsa.

1 Chicken and Avocado Quesadillas

Spread 2 soft tortillas with ¼ cup prepared tomato salsa. Top with 8 oz chopped cooked chicken, 1 sliced avocado, and 1 cup shredded cheddar cheese. Place another tortilla on the top of each. Heat a large skillet until hot, then cook the tortilla sandwiches one at a time for about 5 minutes, turning once, until the tortillas are crisp and the cheese has started to melt. Serve cut into wedges with cucumber and carrot sticks.

2 Avocado and Mozzarella Chicken

Cut 2 boneless, skinless chicken breasts in half horizontally. Season the chicken with a sprinkle of fajita seasoning mix and cook in 2 tablespoons sunflower oil for about 8 minutes, turning once, until golden and cooked through. Top each piece of chicken with 2 slices of tomato, 2–3 slices of avocado and 2 slices of mozzarella cheese. Place the skillet under a preheated medium broiler (keeping the handle away from the heat) for 3–4 minutes, until the cheese melts and starts to brown. Serve with oven fries.

KID-KIDS-XIT

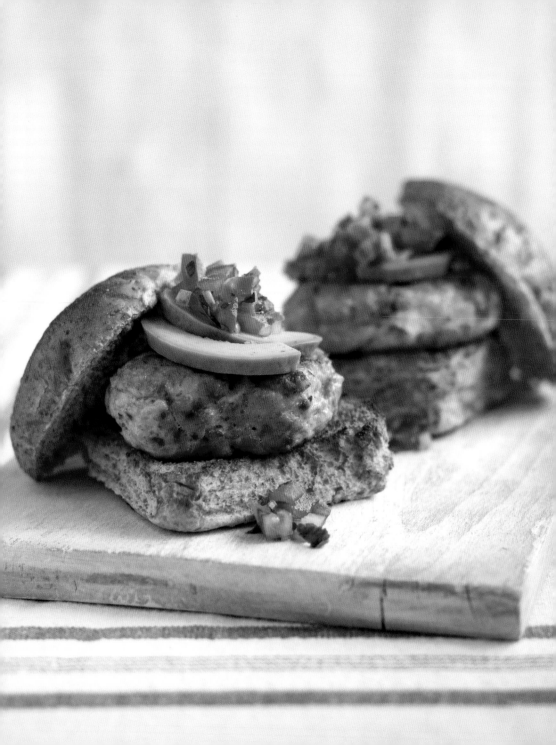

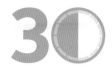 # Easy Ham and Vegetable Pizzas

Makes 4

1⅓ cups all-purpose flour,
   plus extra for dusting
1⅔ cups whole-wheat flour
1 tablespoon demerara sugar
   or other raw sugar
1 teaspoon baking soda
1 cup buttermilk
2 tablespoons olive oil
1 red bell pepper, cored, seeded,
   and cut into strips
1 large zucchini, sliced diagonally
⅔ cup prepared pizza sauce
handful of spinach leaves
4 oz wafer-thin ham
10 oz mozzarella cheese,
   drained and sliced

- Place both flours in a large bowl with the sugar and baking soda and mix well. Add the buttermilk and mix well to form a dough. Turn out onto a floured surface and knead briefly. Divide the dough into 4 pieces, then roll out each piece to about a 6 inch thin circle and place on 2 baking sheets.

- Heat the oil in a large skillet and sauté the bell pepper and zucchini over high heat for 5 minutes.

- Meanwhile, spread each pizza crust with 3–4 tablespoons of the pizza sauce to within 1 inch of the edge. Top each with spinach, ham, zucchini, and bell pepper, then arrange the mozzarella slices over the top.

- Bake at the top of a preheated oven, at 425°F, for 10–12 minutes, until golden and the top is melted.

Simple Ham and Roasted Pepper

Melts Cut 4 prepared cheese biscuits in half and place in a shallow gratin dish. Drain 1 (12 oz) jar mixed roasted peppers, then coarsely chop, mix with 2 handfuls of spinach leaves, and sprinkle over the biscuits. Arrange 4 oz coarsely chopped wafer-thin ham on top, then sprinkle with ⅓ cup grated mozzarella cheese. Cook under a preheated hot broiler for 4–5 minutes and spoon onto serving plates.

Zucchini, Ham, and Bell Pepper Pizzas

Place 4 prepared pizza crusts on 2 baking sheets, spread each with 3 tablespoons prepared pizza sauce, and set aside. Heat 2 tablespoons olive oil in a skillet and cook 1 each small cored, seeded, and coarsely chopped red and yellow bell pepper and 1 thinly sliced zucchini over high heat for 5 minutes, until softened and slightly golden in places. Arrange over the pizza crusts with a handful of spinach leaves and 4 oz wafer-thin ham, then top each with 2 tablespoons grated mozzarella cheese. Bake in a preheated oven, at 425°F, for 10 minutes, until the topping is golden and melted.

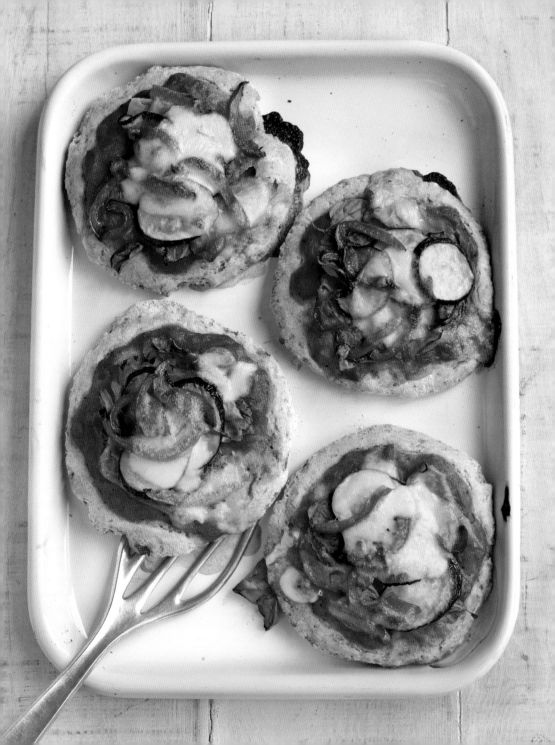

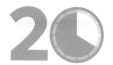

Creamy Chicken, Mushroom, and Broccoli Pasta Gratin

Serves 4

8 oz pasta shapes

3 cups broccoli florets

2 tablespoons olive oil

8 oz skinless, boneless chicken breasts, cut into thin strips

3 cups thickly sliced or quartered cremini mushrooms

1¾ cups crème fraîche or single cream

1 tablespoon Dijon mustard

¼ cups whole-wheat bread crumbs

¼ cup grated Parmesan cheese

mache or green salad, to serve

- Cook the pasta in a large saucepan of lightly salted boiling water according to the package directions. Add the broccoli for the final 5 minutes of the pasta cooking time.

- Meanwhile, heat the oil in a large, heavy skillet and cook the chicken over high heat for 5 minutes. Add the mushrooms and cook for another 3–4 minutes, until both are golden and cooked. Add the crème fraîche or cream and mustard and heat, stirring for 1 minute, until mixed together well.

- Drain the pasta and broccoli well, toss into the skillet, and stir. Transfer to a large gratin dish, sprinkle with the bread crumbs and Parmesan, and cook under a preheated hot broiler for 2–3 minutes, until golden and bubbling.

- Serve with mache or a simple green salad.

Creamy Chicken and Mushroom

Pasta Cook 12 oz pasta shapes in a large saucepan of lightly salted boiling water according to the package directions. Meanwhile, heat 2 tablespoons olive oil in a skillet and cook 8 oz thinly sliced chicken breast and 3 cups quartered cremini mushrooms over high heat for 8 minutes, until golden and cooked through. Add 1¾ cups crème fraîche or single cream and 1 tablespoon Dijon mustard and heat for 1 minute. Drain the pasta, add it to the skillet, and toss before serving.

Chicken, Mushroom, and Broccoli Pasta Gratin

Cook 8 oz pasta shapes in a large saucepan of lightly salted boiling water according to the package directions, adding 3½ cups broccoli florets for the final 5 minutes. Drain. In a separate skillet, heat 2 tablespoons olive oil and cook 8 oz thinly sliced chicken breast over high heat for 8–10 minutes, until golden and cooked through. Meanwhile, heat 4 tablespoons butter in a large, heavy skillet and cook 3 cups coarsely chopped mushrooms over high heat for 5 minutes, until golden.

Add 2 tablespoons all-purpose flour and stir well to mix, then return to the heat for 30 seconds, stirring. Remove from the heat and add 1¼ cups milk, a little at a time, stirring well between each addition until smooth. Return to the heat and bring to a boil, stirring well until boiled and thickened. Add 1¾ cups crème fraîche or single cream, then mix with the pasta, broccoli, and chicken. Pile into a large gratin dish and top with ¼ cup whole-wheat bread crumbs mixed with ¼ cup grated Parmesan cheese. Cook under a preheated broiler for 3–4 minutes, until golden and bubbling.

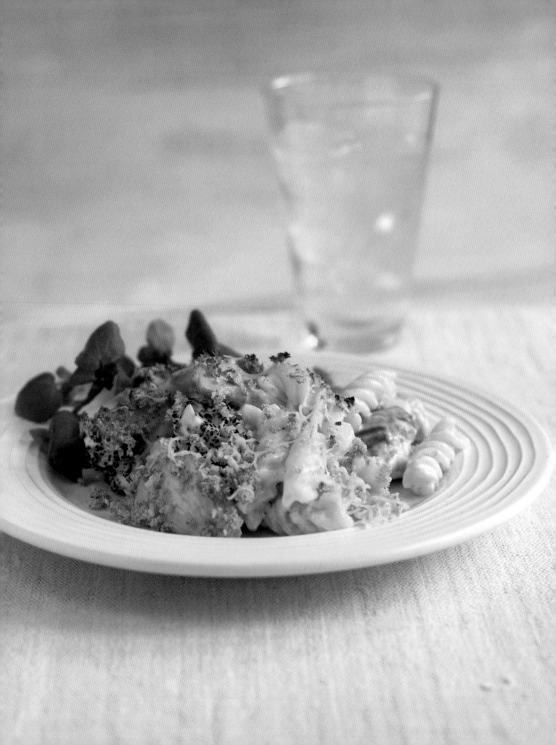

30 Lamb Casserole (with Hidden Veg!)

Serves 4

3 sweet potatoes, cut into coarse chunks

3 carrots, peeled and cut into chunks, plus 1 large carrot, peeled and shredded

12 oz ground lamb or turkey

1 zucchini, shredded

1 beef bouillon cube (or chicken bouillon cube if using turkey), crumbled

1 (14½ oz) can diced tomatoes

¼ cup Worcestershire sauce

3 tablespoons tomato paste

2 tablespoons butter

¼ cup grated Parmesan cheese

green vegetables, to serve

- Cook the sweet potato and carrot chunks in a large saucepan of lightly salted boiling water for 15–20 minutes, until tender.

- Meanwhile, heat a large skillet for 1 minute. Add the ground meat and dry-fry over high heat for 5 minutes, until browned, stirring frequently. Add the shredded carrot and zucchini and cook for 3 minutes, then add the bouillon cube, tomatoes, Worcestershire sauce, and tomato paste. Stir well, then bring to a boil. Reduce the heat, cover, and simmer for 10 minutes.

- Drain the sweet potatoes and carrots, add the butter, and mash well using a potato masher or electric mixer until thick and almost smooth.

- Spoon the meat into a shallow gratin dish and spoon the mashed vegetables over the top. Sprinkle with the Parmesan and cook under a preheated broiler for 3–4 minutes, until golden. Serve hot with green vegetables.

---

10 Minute Steaks with Vegetable Sauce

Season four (4 oz) minute steaks with a little black pepper. Heat 2 tablespoons olive oil in a large skillet and cook 1 small coarsely chopped zucchini and 1 small, peeled and coarsely chopped carrot for 5 minutes. Meanwhile, cook the steaks under a hot broiler for 2–3 minutes on each side. Add 1 (14½ oz) can diced tomatoes and 1 tablespoon tomato paste to the vegetables and stir and cook for 2 minutes. Serve the steaks with the sauce spooned over them.

20 Hidden-Vegetable Meat Sauce with Mashed Sweet Potatoes

Cook 3 coarsely chopped sweet potatoes in a saucepan of lightly salted boiling water for 15 minutes, until tender. Heat a large, heavy skillet for 1 minute. Add 1 lb ground round beef or ground sirloin beef and cook over high heat for 5 minutes, until browned. Add 1 trimmed and shredded zucchini and 1 peeled and shredded carrot and cook for another 2 minutes. Add 1 tablespoon tomato paste and 2 tablespoons Worcestershire sauce and cook, stirring, for 2 minutes. Add 1 beef bouillon cube and 1¼ cups water, bring to a boil, and cook for 5 minutes. Blend 1 tablespoon cornstarch with 2 tablespoons water and add to the pan, cooking for 2 minutes and stirring until thickened. Drain the sweet potatoes and mash with 2 tablespoons butter. Serve spooned onto warmed serving plates with a ladleful of meat with the sauce.

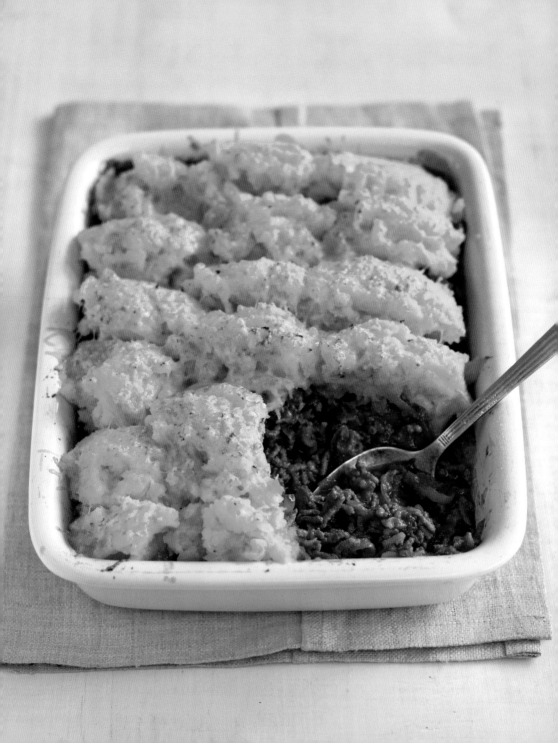

30 Pork Cutlets with Tomato Pasta

Serves 4

2 (6 oz) boneless pork cutlets,
  each cut into 2 thinner pieces
2 eggs, beaten
1 cup bread crumbs
12 oz spaghetti
1 small onion, chopped
1 garlic clove, crushed
5 ripe tomatoes, chopped
½ teaspoon granulated sugar
small handful of basil leaves, torn
3 tablespoons sunflower oil
salt and black pepper
grated cheese, to serve

- Place the cutlet pieces between sheets of plastic wrap and bash with a rolling pin until ⅛–¼ inch thick. Place the beaten eggs on one plate and the bread crumbs on another and season well. Dip the pork in the egg to coat, then the bread crumbs, pressing firmly to coat.

- Cook the spaghetti in a saucepan of lightly salted boiling water according to the package directions, until just tender.

- Heat 1 tablespoon of the oil in a skillet, add the onion and garlic, and cook for 5 minutes, until softened. Add the tomatoes and sugar and season with salt and black pepper. Cook for about 5 minutes, until the tomatoes are soft and pulpy. Stir in the basil.

- Meanwhile heat the remaining oil in a large skillet, add the pork cutlets, and cook, in batches, 2 at a time for 3 minutes on each side, until golden, crisp and cooked through.

- Drain the spaghetti, mix with the tomato sauce, sprinkle with grated cheese, and serve with the pork cutlets.

1 Pork and Cherry Tomato Stir-Fry

Cut 4 (4 oz) boneless pork cutlets into strips and stir-fry in 2 tablespoons sunflower oil over high heat for 2 minutes. Add 8 cherry tomatoes and stir-fry for 1 minute, then stir in 1½ cups prepared tomato and herb sauce and 1 cup cooked rice. Stir well and heat through until piping hot. Serve with crusty bread.

2 Pan-Fried Pork with Creamy

Tomato Sauce Thickly slice 1 lb pork tenderloin and cook in 2 tablespoons olive oil for about 5 minutes, turning once, until browned and cooked through. Remove from the saucepan and set aside. Add 1 crushed garlic clove, 1¼ cups tomato puree, and ½ cup mascarpone cheese to the pan. Bring to a boil, stirring, then season with salt and black pepper and return the pork to the pan. Heat through for a few minutes, then serve with peas and oven fries or potato wedges.

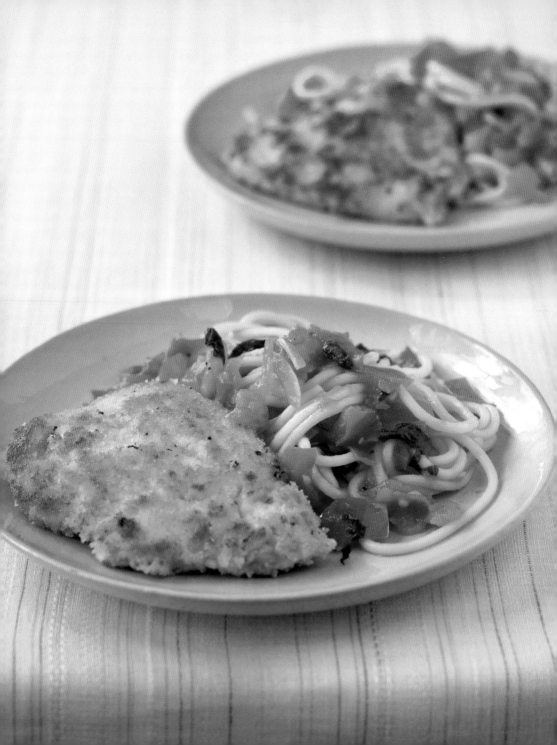

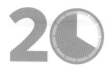

Corn Fritters with Tomato Salsa

Makes 16

1 cup all-purpose flour
1 egg
⅔ cup milk
1 (11 oz) can corn kernels, drained
¼ cup sunflower oil
salt and black pepper
prepared guacamole, to serve

For the salsa

3 ripe tomatoes, chopped
2 scallions, chopped
pinch of granulated sugar
2 tablespoons prepared
  French dressing

- Place the flour in a bowl, make a well in the center, and break in the egg. Gradually add the milk, mixing with a hand whisk to make a smooth, thick batter. Season with salt and black pepper and stir in the corn kernels.

- Heat the oil in a large skillet, add spoonfuls of the batter, and cook, in batches, for about 5 minutes, turning once, until golden and crisp. Drain on paper towels.

- To make the salsa, place the tomatoes in a bowl and crush lightly with a fork. Add the scallions, sugar, and French dressing, season with salt and black pepper, and mix well.

- Serve the fritters with the tomato salsa and guacamole.

 Corn and Mixed Bean Tacos

Mix together 1 (8¾ oz) can corn kernels, drained, and ¾ cup each rinsed and drained, canned kidney beans and black beans with a pinch of chili pepper in a bowl. Spoon into 4 taco shells with ¼ shredded iceberg lettuce, 2 shredded carrots, and a little shredded cheese. Serve with tomato salsa and sour cream.

 Corn, Bacon, and Cheese Tarts

Cook 4 bacon slices under a preheated hot broiler until crisp, then chop and set aside. Unroll 1 sheet of ready-to-bake puff pastry, cut into 4 equal squares, and place on a baking sheet lined with parchment paper. Mix together 1½ cups prepared cheese sauce, 1 (8¾ oz) can corn kernels, drained, and the chopped cooked bacon. Spoon the mixture onto the pastry squares and spread evenly, leaving a ½ inch border at the edge. Sprinkle with ½ cup shredded cheddar cheese and bake in a preheated oven, at 400°F, for 15–20 minutes, until well risen and golden. Serve warm with salad.

KID-KIDS-GAD

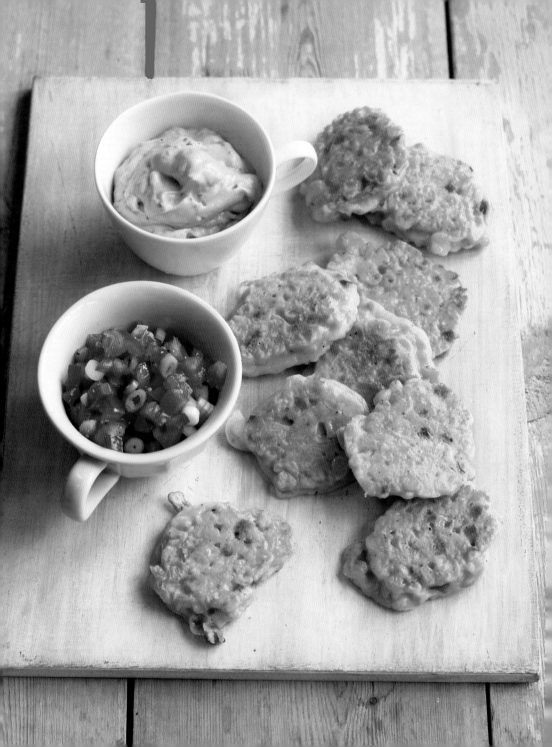

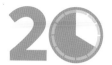 # Singapore Noodles

Serves 4

2 tablespoons dark soy sauce
1 teaspoon light brown sugar
¼ cup water
8 oz thin rice noodles
3 tablespoons sunflower oil
2 eggs, lightly beaten
1 onion, finely sliced
1 green bell pepper, cored,
  seeded, and cut into strips
8 oz cooked, peeled shrimp,
  defrosted if frozen
1 inch piece of fresh ginger root,
  peeled and grated
2 teaspoons curry powder
½ small cabbage, finely shredded
salt and black pepper

- In a small bowl, mix together the soy sauce, sugar, and measured water and set aside.

- Soak the noodles in boiling water for 2 minutes to soften, then drain well.

- Heat 1 tablespoon of the oil in a wok or large skillet. Add the beaten eggs, season with salt and black pepper, and cook, stirring, for 1–2 minutes, until a flat omelet is formed. Remove from the wok, cut into strips, and set aside.

- Heat the remaining oil in the wok, add the onion and green bell pepper, and stir-fry for 2 minutes to soften. Add the shrimp, ginger, curry powder, and cabbage and cook for another 2 minutes.

- Stir in the soy sauce mixture and noodles and heat through. Add the scrambled egg and lightly stir through. Serve in bowls and top with the egg strips.

1⃝ Shrimp and Pea Noodles

Prepare 4 oz egg noodles according to the the package directions. Meanwhile, sauté 3 cups button mushrooms, halved if large, ⅔ cup frozen peas, and 8 oz peeled shrimp, defrosted if frozen, for about 3 minutes, until the mushrooms are browned and the peas are cooked. Stir into the noodles and serve with a dash of soy sauce.

3⃝ Singapore Noodle Stir-Fry

Place 8 oz cooked, peeled shrimp, defrosted if frozen, in a shallow dish. Pour a mixture of 2 tablespoons dark soy sauce, 1 teaspoon light brown sugar, 1 inch piece of fresh ginger root, peeled and grated, 2 teaspoons curry powder, and ¼ cup water over the shrimp. Mix well and set aside for 15 minutes. Meanwhile, prepare 8 oz thin rice noodles according to the

package directions, then drain. Heat 2 tablespoons sunflower oil in a wok or large skillet. Add 1 sliced onion and 1 green bell pepper, cored, seeded, and cut into strips, and stir-fry for 5 minutes, until softened. Remove the shrimp from the marinade (reserving the marinade), add to the wok, and stir-fry for 2 minutes, then stir in the reserved marinade and bring to a boil. Add the noodles, toss lightly to mix, and heat through.

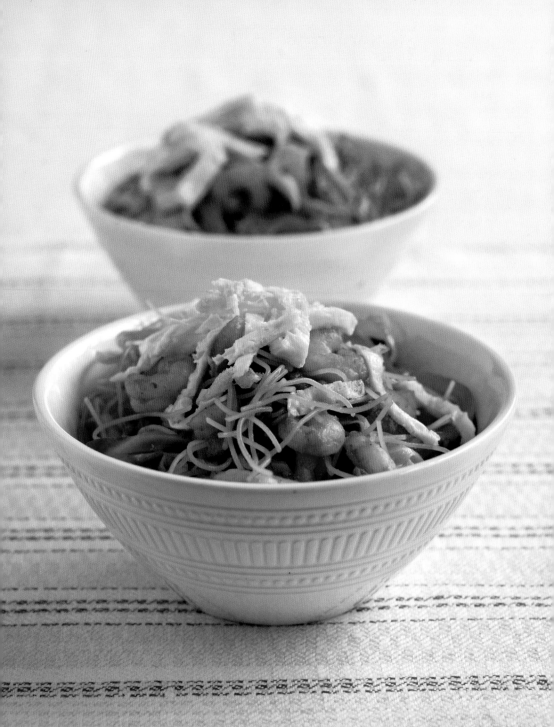

30 Fish Sticks with Sweet Potato Fries

Serves 4

4 sweet potatoes, cut into
  slim wedges

2 tablespoons olive oil

1 lb cod fillets, cut into
  1 inch strips

1 cup all-purpose flour

1¾ cups whole-wheat
  bread crumbs

3 tablespoons chopped parsley,
  plus extra to garnish (optional)

2 eggs, beaten

salt and black pepper

tartar sauce, to serve

- Place the sweet potato wedges in a bowl with the oil and toss well to coat, then season with a little salt and black pepper. Transfer to a baking sheet and cook in a preheated oven, at 400°F, for 20 minutes.

- Meanwhile, toss the fish strips in the flour. Place the bread crumbs in a bowl, add the parsley, and toss well. Working quickly, take a floured fish strip and dip in the egg, then in the herbed bread crumbs, and place on a baking sheet. Continue until all are used, then bake in the oven for 15 minutes, until the bread crumbs are golden and the fish is opaque and cooked through.

- Serve with the sweet potato wedges and tartar sauce, with parsley.

---

1 Fish Sticks with Mashed Sweet Potatoes

Bring a saucepan of lightly salted water to a boil. Peel 3 sweet potatoes and coarsely chop into small pieces. Add to the pan and cook for 8 minutes. Meanwhile, cook 8 frozen fish sticks under a preheated hot broiler for 6–7 minutes, turning once, until golden and cooked through. Drain the potatoes and add 2 tablespoons butter. Coarsely mash with a potato masher. Stir in 2 tablespoons chopped parsley and season with black pepper. Spoon onto warmed serving plates and serve with the fish sticks.

2 Roasted Sweet Potatoes and Cod with a Crunchy Topping

Cut 2 sweet potatoes into small cubes. Place in a roasting pan, drizzle with 2 tablespoons olive oil, and toss well to coat. Roast in the top of a preheated oven, at 425°F, for 15–18 minutes. Meanwhile, place 4 (4 oz) small cod fillets on a separate roasting pan and season generously with black pepper. Mix 2 tablespoons whole-wheat bread crumbs with 1 tablespoon chopped parsley and sprinkle over the fish. Roast in the oven with the potatoes for 10–12 minutes, until the fish is opaque and cooked through and the bread crumbs have turned golden and crunchy in places. Serve with the sweet potato cubes with spoonfuls of tartar sauce or mayonnaise, if desired.

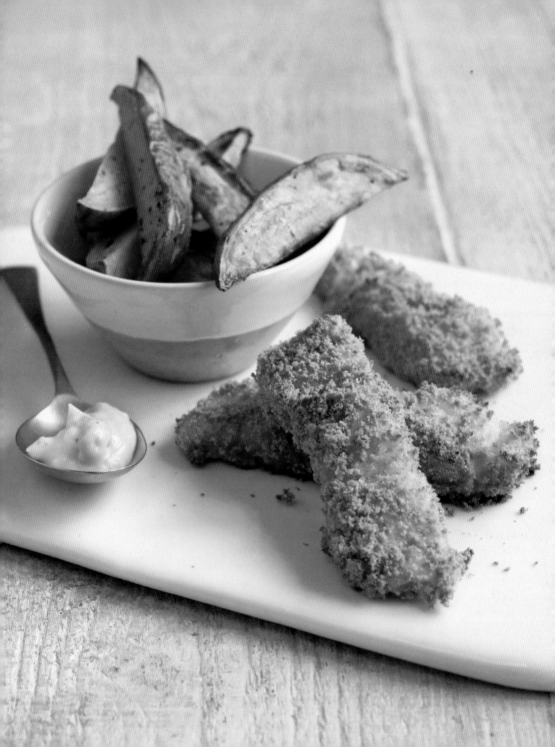

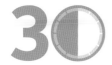

Sausage, Zucchini, and Tomato Risotto

Serves 4

4 thick pork sausages
2 tablespoon olive oil
1 onion, chopped
1 zucchini, chopped
1 cup (isotto rice
1 (14½ oz) can diced tomatoes
3 cups hot chicken stock
½ cup grated Parmesan cheese,
  plus extra to serve
salt and black pepper
garlic bread, to serve

- Cook the sausages under a preheated broiler for 10 minutes, turning occasionally, until browned and cooked through.

- Meanwhile, heat the oil in a large, deep skillet or shallow saucepan. Add the onion and zucchini and sauté for 5 minutes to soften. Add the rice and stir well. Stir in the tomatoes and half the stock. Bring to a boil, stirring occasionally, and simmer until almost all the stock has been absorbed. Add the remaining stock and simmer, stirring occasionally, until the rice is tender and the stock has been absorbed.

- Slice the cooked sausages and stir into the risotto with the Parmesan. Season with salt and black pepper and serve with extra Parmesan and garlic bread.

Sausage and Zucchini Ciabatta Pizzas Cut a ciabatta loaf in half horizontally, place on a baking sheet and spread the cut sides with 3 tablespoons prepared pizza sauce. Chop 12 cooked small sausages and sprinkle them over the tops with ½ thinly sliced zucchini. Sprinkle with 1 cup grated mozzarella cheese and bake in a preheated oven, at 425°F, for 8 minutes, until the cheese has melted and bread is crisp.

Sausage, Zucchini, and Tomato Kebabs Cut 8 small sausages into thirds and thread onto skewers alternately with 8 cherry tomatoes and 1 thickly sliced zucchini. Brush with some prepared barbecue sauce and cook under a preheated broiler for about 10 minutes, turning occasionally, until the sausages are cooked and the zucchini is tender. Serve with rice, corn, and extra barbecue sauce.

KID-KIDS-LAK

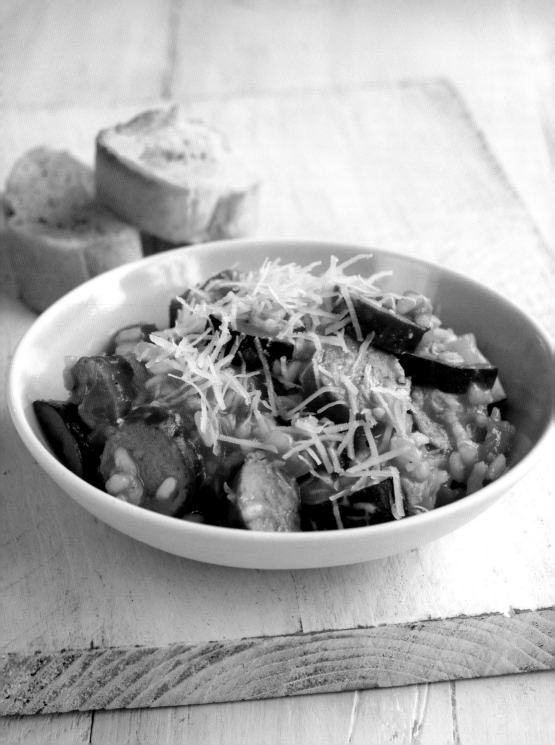

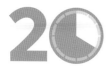

Cabbage Potato Cakes

Makes 8

2 tablespoons olive oil

1 red onion, finely sliced

2 cups shredded savoy or
green cabbage

2 cups prepared mashed potatoes

1 tablespoon Dijon mustard

¼ cup finely grated Gruyère
cheese or Swiss cheese

1 egg yolk

⅔ cup seasoned flour

¼ cup vegetable oil

rich tomato sauce, to serve

- Heat the olive oil in a large, heavy skillet and cook the onion over medium heat for 3 minutes, until beginning to soften. Add the cabbage and cook, stirring, for another 3–4 minutes, until softened and beginning to turn golden.

- Place the mashed potatoes in a large mixing bowl, add the Dijon mustard and cheese, and mix well, then add the egg yolk and mix again. Add the warm cabbage-and-onion mixture and stir again, then divide the mixture into 8 pieces. Shape into patties using floured hands, then dip each one in a little seasoned flour and set aside.

- Heat the vegetable oil in a large, heavy skillet and cook the patties over medium heat for 2–3 minutes on each side until golden. Serve hot with rich tomato sauce.

Potato and Cabbage Soup

Place 3 cups shredded savoy or green cabbage in a saucepan with 2½ cups chicken or vegetable stock and bring to a boil. Add 1¼ cups chilled prepared mashed potatoes and 1 tablespoon Dijon mustard and cook, stirring, for another 5 minutes. Transfer the mixture to a food processor and proces until smooth. Serve in warmed serving bowls with croutons and sprinkled with grated cheese.

Cheesy Cabbage Potato Cakes

Heat ¼ cup olive oil and 1 tablespoon butter in a large, heavy skillet and cook 1 sliced red onion for 5 minutes, until softened and golden. Add 2½ cups chilled prepared mashed potatoes and cook over high heat for 10 minutes, stirring occasionally, until golden and crisp in places but not burning. Add 3 cups shredded savoy or green cabbage and cook for another 6–7 minutes, until softened, stirring occasionally. Sprinkle with 1 cup shredded cheddar cheese. Place the skillet under a preheated hot broiler, keeping the handle away from the heat, and cook for 5 minutes, until golden. Serve in wedges.

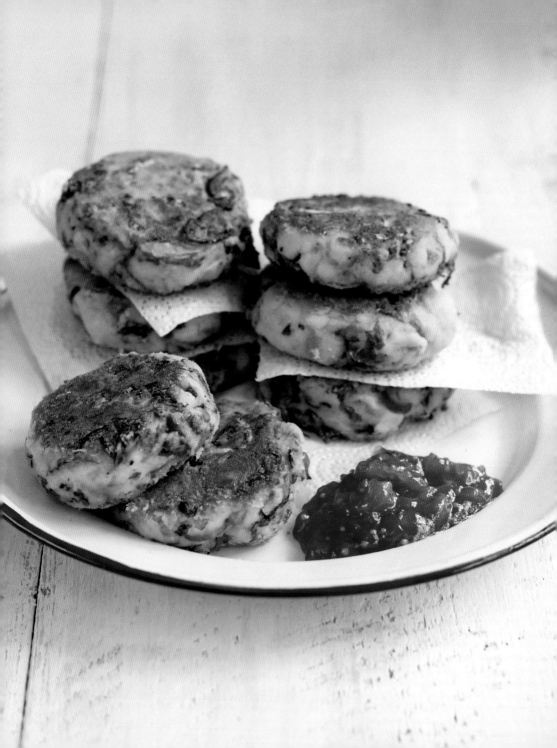

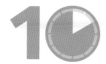 # Creamy Garlic Mushroom Bagels

Serves 2

1 tablespoon olive oil

2 cups button mushrooms, halved if large

⅓ cup garlic and herb cream cheese

2–3 tablespoons milk

2 bagels

½ cup shredded cheddar cheese, to serve

- Heat the oil in a skillet. Add the mushrooms and cook over high heat for 3–4 minutes, until golden and tender. Reduce the heat and stir in the cream cheese and milk to make a creamy sauce, adding a little more milk, if necessary.

- Meanwhile, halve and toast the bagels under a preheated broiler. Spoon the creamy mushrooms on top and sprinkle with the cheddar cheese to serve.

 Creamy Mushroom Soup with Garlic Bagel Toasts Sauté 1 small chopped onion and 4 cups (8 oz) chopped mushrooms in 2 tablespoons butter for 5 minutes, until the onion has softened. Pour in 1¼ cups vegetable stock, season with salt and black pepper, and simmer for 5 minutes. Blend with a handheld blender until almost smooth, stir in ½ cup crème fraîche or single cream, and reheat. Spread the halved bagels with prepared garlic butter and broil until golden and crisp. Serve the soup with a spoonful of crème fraîche and the toasted garlic bagels.

 Baked Garlicky Mozzarella Mushrooms Sauté 1 small onion and 3 chopped bacon slices in 1 tablespoon olive oil for 5 minutes, until the onion softens and the bacon is crisp. Add 1 crushed garlic clove and 2 slices of bread, cut into small cubes, and cook for 2 minutes, then remove from the heat and stir in 2 tablespoons chopped parsley. Place 3 cups open-cup mushrooms in a baking dish. Sprinkle the onion mixture over the top, sprinkle with 5 oz chopped mozzarella cheese, and drizzle with olive oil. Bake in a preheated oven, at 400°F, for 20 minutes, until the cheese is melted and golden and the mushrooms are cooked. Serve with salad.

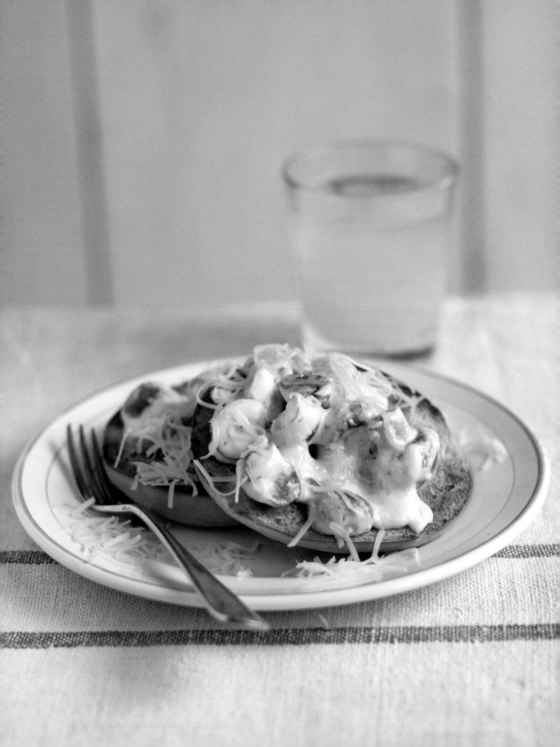

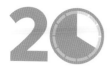

Hidden Vegetable Pasta

Serves 4

1 tablespoon olive oil
1 onion, chopped
2 carrots, chopped
½ small butternut squash, chopped
1 leek, rinsed, trimmed and chopped
1 zucchini, chopped
2 cups chopped mushrooms
2 cups tomato puree or tomato sauce with garlic and herbs
⅔ cup vegetable stock
12 oz linguine or tagliatelle
salt and black pepper
grated cheese, to serve

- Heat the oil in a large saucepan. Add the onion, carrots, butternut squash, leek, zucchini, and mushrooms and cook over high heat for 5 minutes to soften.

- Add the tomato puree or sauce and stock, bring to a boil, then reduce the heat, cover, and simmer for 10 minutes. Meanwhile, cook the linguine or tagliatelle in a large saucepan of lightly salted boiling water according to the package directions, until tender, then drain and return to the pan.

- Using a handheld blender or food processor, blend the sauce until smooth, adding a little water, if necessary. Season with salt and black pepper, then toss with the linguine or tagliatelle. Serve with plenty of grated cheese.

Quick Vegetable Tortelloni Gratin

Cook 1 (11 oz) package spinach and ricotta tortelloni in a saucepan of lightly salted boiling water for 3–4 minutes, then drain. Meanwhile, heat 1½ cups prepared tomato sauce in a saucepan. Add ½ coarsely grated zucchini, 1 peeled and shredded carrot, and 1 cup chopped mushrooms and cook for 5 minutes to soften the vegetables. Mix together the tortelloni and sauce, transfer to a heatproof dish, and top with 5 oz sliced mozzarella cheese. Place under a preheated hot broiler for 2–3 minutes, until the cheese is bubbling.

Hidden Vegetable Pizzas

Heat 1 tablespoon olive oil in a large saucepan, add 1 small chopped onion, 1 peeled and chopped carrot, ¼ peeled and chopped butternut squash, 1 chopped zucchini, and 1 cup chopped mushrooms. Cook, stirring, for 5 minutes to soften, then add 1 (14½ oz) can diced tomatoes with garlic and herbs. Bring to a boil, cover, and simmer for 10 minutes. Blend until smooth with a handheld blender or food processor and season with salt and black pepper. Spread the sauce onto 4 prepared pizza crusts, top with 5 oz sliced mozzarella cheese, and bake in a preheated oven, at 425°F, for 10 minutes, until the cheese has melted and is starting to brown and the crusts are crisp. Serve with salad.

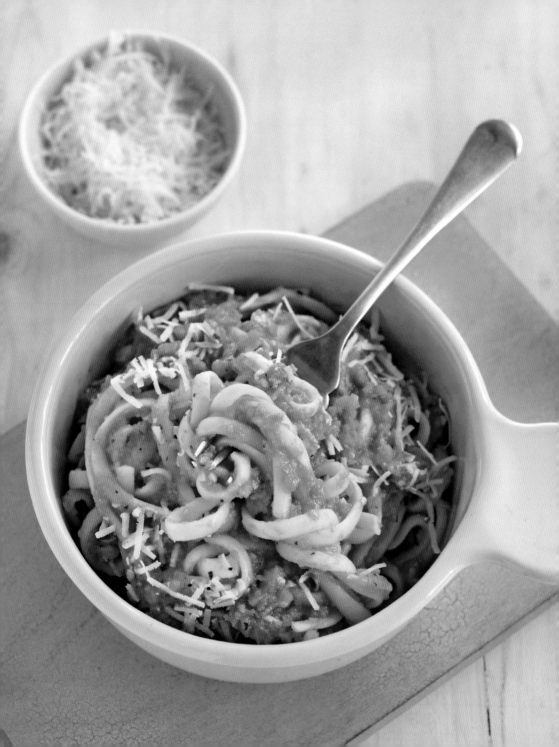

30 Chicken Nuggets with Sun-Dried Tomato Sauce

Serves 4

⅓ cup whole-wheat flour
½ teaspoon ground cumin
½ teaspoon ground coriander
½ teaspoon paprika
2 eggs, beaten
2 tablespoons olive oil
1 lb chicken breasts cut into
   1½ in chunks
black pepper

For the sauce

1½ cups drained sun-dried
   tomatoes, drained
1 small tomato, halved and seeded
2 tablespoons mayonnaise

- Mix together the flour, cumin, coriander, and paprika and season with black pepper. Divide between 2 plates. Put the beaten egg on a separate plate.

- Pour the oil onto a large baking sheet and heat in a preheated oven, at 400°F, for 5 minutes.

- Meanwhile, one piece at a time, toss the chicken in the first plate of flour, then coat in the egg and then in the second plate of flour. Remove the baking sheet from the oven and toss the nuggets in the oil. Return to the oven and roast for 20 minutes, until golden and crisp.

- Meanwhile, to make the sun-dried tomato sauce, place both kinds of tomato in a food processor with the mayonnaise and blend until smooth. Remove the nuggets from the oven, drain on paper towels, and serve with the tomato sauce.

 Spiced Chicken and Sun-Dried Tomato Pita Breads Cut 12 oz boneless, skinless chicken breasts into thin strips and toss with ½ teaspoon each ground cumin, ground coriander, and paprika. Heat 1 tablespoon olive oil in a skillet and cook the chicken for 7–8 minutes, until golden and cooked through, adding 6 coarsely chopped sun-dried tomatoes for the final minute. Meanwhile, take 4 small pita breads and lightly toast. Cut open, using a serrated knife, and fill with salad and the hot chicken and tomato mixture. Serve warm.

 Sun-Dried Tomato and Spiced Chicken Skewers Cut 3 (5 oz) chicken breasts into (1 inch) chunks, then place in a bowl and toss with ½ teaspoon ground cumin, ½ teaspoon ground coriander, and ½ teaspoon paprika. Thread onto 8 presoaked wooden skewers (for 30 minutes) or metal skewers, adding 2 sun-dried tomatoes and 1 cherry tomato to each skewer. Cook under a preheated medium broiler for 8–10 minutes, turning once, until the chicken is cooked and the tomatoes soft. Serve sprinkled with chopped parsley and ketchup.

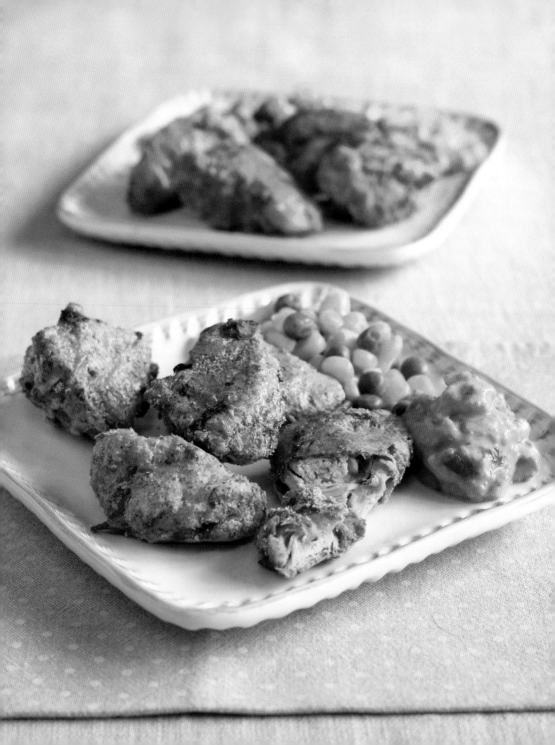

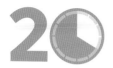

Bacon, Pea, and Potato Frittata

Serves 4

2 tablespoons olive oil
2 potatoes, cut into small cubes
6 bacon slices, coarsely chopped
1 cup frozen peas
⅓ cup cold water
6 eggs
1 teaspoon Dijon mustard
black pepper
crusty bread, to serve

- Heat the oil in a medium, heavy skillet and cook the potatoes over high heat for 3–4 minutes, until golden in places. Add the bacon and cook for another 5 minutes, until golden, stirring occasionally. Add the peas and the measured water and bring to a boil. Cover with a baking sheet and cook for another 2–3 minutes.

- Meanwhile, beat the eggs with the mustard and season generously with black pepper.

- Remove the baking sheet from the top of the skillet, pour in the eggs, and mix well to evenly distribute the filling and make sure any surplus water mixes with the eggs. Cook for 2–3 minutes, until the bottom is set, then place the skillet under a preheated broiler (keeping the handle away from the heat) and cook for another 2 minutes, until the top is golden and set.

- Serve in wedges with crusty bread.

Bacon and Pea Omelet

Heat 1 tablespoon olive oil in a medium, heavy skillet and cook 4 coarsely chopped bacon slices over high heat for 3 minutes, until crisp. Add ½ cup frozen peas and cook for another 1 minute. Meanwhile, beat 4 eggs in a small small bowl, season with black pepper, and pour into the skillet. Gently cook for 2–3 minutes, until the bottom is set, then place the pan under a preheated broiler (keeping the handle away from the heat) and cook for 1 minute, until the top is set and serve.

Baked Bacon, Pea, and Red Pepper Tortilla

Heat 2 tablespoons olive oil in a skillet and cook 6 coarsely chopped bacon slices with 1 chopped onion and 1 cored, seeded, and chopped red bell pepper for 5 minutes. Add 3 coarsely chopped tomatoes and 1 cup frozen peas and stir and cook for 1 minute, then transfer into a mixing bowl. Beat 8 eggs in a separate small bowl, season well with black pepper, pour into the vegetables, and mix well.

Lightly grease a 7 x 11 inch roasting pan with oil, then pour in the egg and vegetable mixture. Bake in a preheated oven, at 400°F, for 20 minutes, until golden and puffed. Cut into squares to serve.

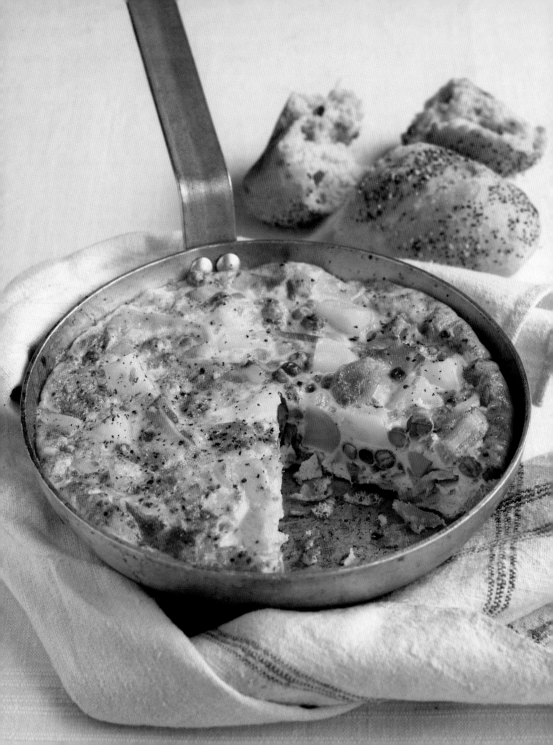

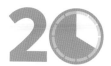

Veggie Noodles with Hoisin Sauce

Serves 4

6 oz egg noodles

¼ cup sesame oil

16 baby corn, coarsely chopped

1 large red bell pepper, cored, seeded, and cut into strips

bunch of scallions, coarsely chopped

2 cups coarsely chopped green beans

1 inch piece of fresh ginger root, peeled and grated

1 garlic clove, crushed

¼ cup honey

1 tablespoon dark soy sauce

¼ cup sweet chili sauce

¼ cup toasted sesame seeds

- Cook the noodles in a large saucepan of lightly salted boiling water according to the package directions.

- Meanwhile, heat the oil in a large, heavy skillet. Add the baby corn and red bell pepper over high heat for 3 minutes, stirring occasionally. Add the scallions, green beans, ginger, and garlic and stir-fry for 4 minutes, until softened, but not too golden—reduce the heat if they start to brown.

- Drain the noodles, add to the skillet, and toss. Mix together the honey, soy sauce, sweet chili sauce, and sesame seeds, pour over the noodles, and toss again for 1 minute, until hot. Serve in warmed serving bowls.

 Quick Veggie Noodles

Heat 2 tablespoons sesame oil in a large wok or skillet and stir-fry 1 (1 lb) package stir-fry vegetables for 3–4 minutes, until tender but retaining their shape. In a separate saucepan, heat 2 tablespoons sesame oil and stir-fry 8 oz straight-to-wok egg noodles for 2–3 minutes, until separated and hot. Toss into the vegetables, add 1 tablespoon dark soy sauce and 2 tablespoons sweet chili sauce, and toss. Sprinkle with 2 tablespoons toasted sesame seeds, toss again, and serve.

 Vegetable and Egg Noodles

Cook 8 oz soba noodles in a saucepan of lightly salted boiling water according to the package directions, until tender, then drain. Meanwhile, heat 2 tablespoons sesame oil in a large wok or skillet. Break in 2 beaten eggs, cook over medium heat for 2 minutes, until golden and set, then flip over and cook for another 30 seconds, until golden. Remove from the wok and coarsely chop, then set aside. Heat another 2 tablespoons sesame oil in the wok or skillet and cook 16 baby corn, cut in half lengthwise, and 1 large red bell pepper, seeded and cut into strips, for 5 minutes. Add a bunch of coarsely chopped scallions, 3 cups coarsely chopped sugarsnap peas, a 1 inch piece of fresh ginger root, peeled and grated, and 1 garlic clove, crushed, and stir-fry for another 3–4 minutes. Add the drained noodles and stir-fry for 2 minutes, add the egg, and toss. Serve hot in warmed serving bowls sprinkled with 2 tablespoons toasted sesame seeds, drizzled with soy sauce or chili sauce, if desired.

KID-KIDS-GOT

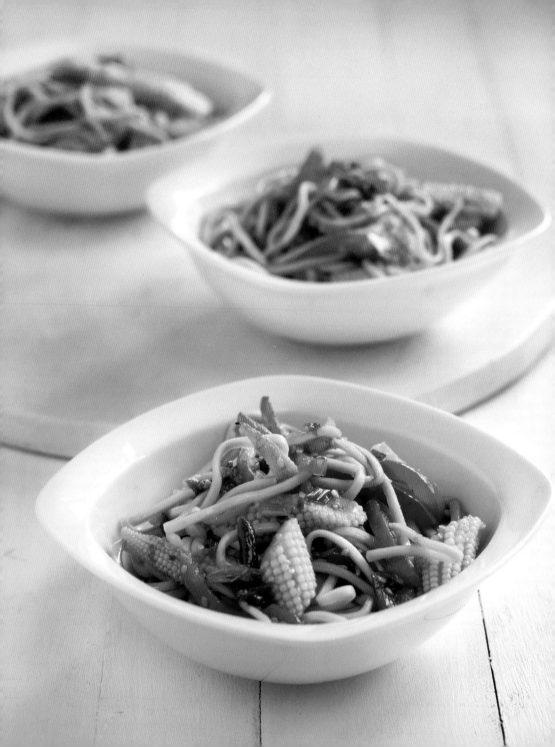

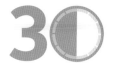

30 Potato Skins with Homemade Guacamole

Serves 4

6 baking potatoes, washed
¼ cup olive oil
1 teaspoon Cajun spice
1 avocado, halved, peeled, and pitted
finely grated rind and juice of ½ lemon
1 tablespoon sweet chili sauce
2 tablespoons finely chopped cilantro
black pepper

- Prick the potatoes all over and cook for 10 minutes in a microwave on full power. Remove from the microwave, cut each in half, and scoop out most of the potato, leaving a ½ inch border of potato next to the skin. Discard the potato flesh (or keep for mashed potatoes for another recipe).

- Cut each half into 2 wedges and place on a baking sheet. Mix the oil with the Cajun spice and brush over the potato skins on both sides. Place on a baking sheet and cook under a preheated broiler for 5–7 minutes, then turn the skins over and cook for another 5–7 minutes, until crisp and golden.

- Meanwhile, mash the avocado with the lemon rind and juice, season with black pepper, and mix in the chili sauce and cilantro. Transfer to a small serving bowl and put it on a serving platter. Place the hot potato skins on the platter and use them to dip into the guacamole.

 Pan-Fried Potato Cakes with Guacamole Divide 1½ cups chilled prepared mashed potatoes into 4. Shape each portion into 4 patty shapes and toss in seasoned flour. Heat ¼ cup vegetable oil in a large, heavy skillet and cook the potato cakes over high heat for 4 minutes on each side, until golden. Serve hot with spoonfuls of chilled prepared guacamole and sprinkle with 2 finely chopped scallions to serve.

 Potato Wedges with Guacamole Place 1 lb prepared herbed potato wedges in a roasting pan. Cook under a preheated broiler for 8–10 minutes, until golden, then turn them over using a spatula and cook for another 6–8 minutes, until golden and crisp. Meanwhile, make the guacamole. Mash 1 peeled, pitted ripe avocado with the finely grated rind and juice of 1 lemon, then stir in 1 tablespoon sweet chili sauce and 2 tablespoons chopped cilantro. Serve the hot wedges sprinkled with 2 finely chopped scallions ready to dip in the guacamole.

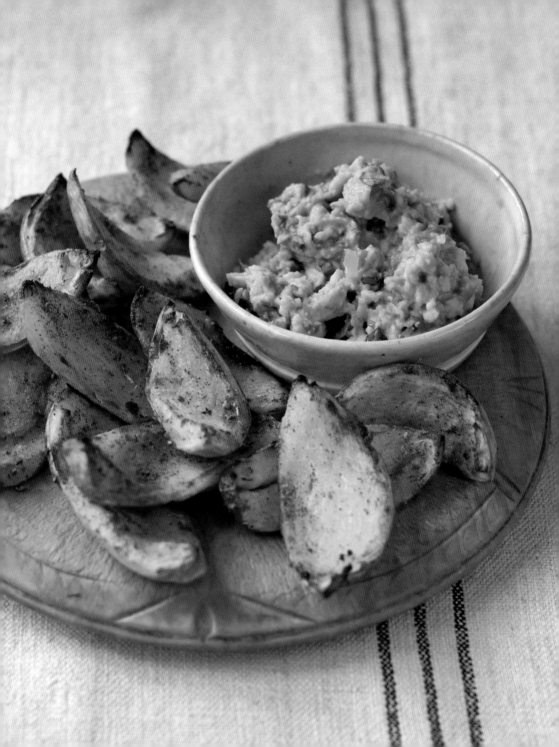

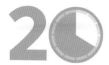

Tomato and Spinach Ravioli Gratin

Serves 4

1 (11 oz) package spinach
and ricotta ravioli

3 tablespoons olive oil

16 cherry tomatoes

2 (14½ oz) cans diced tomatoes

3 tablespoons sun-dried
tomato paste

1 (6 oz) package baby spinach
leaves

5 oz mozzarella cheese, drained
and thinly sliced

¼ cup grated Parmesan cheese

black pepper

To serve

garlic bread

salad

- Cook the ravioli in a large saucepan of lightly salted boiling water according to the package directions, then drain.

- Meanwhile, heat the oil in a large, heavy skillet, add the cherry tomatoes to the skillet, and cook for 3–4 minutes, until beginning to soften and "pop." Add the diced tomatoes and sun-dried tomato paste and bring to a boil, then add the baby spinach leaves and cook and stir for 3–4 minutes, until all the ingredients are piping hot and the spinach has wilted. Season generously with black pepper.

- Add the drained pasta to the skillet and toss well, then transfer to a shallow gratin dish. Arrange the mozzarella slices over the pasta, then sprinkle with the Parmesan.

- Cook under a preheated broiler for 3–4 minutes, until golden and bubbling. Serve with garlic bread and salad.

Spinach Ravioli with Tomato Sauce

Cook 1 (11 oz) package spinach and ricotta ravioli in lightly salted boiling water according to the package directions, then drain. Meanwhile, heat 1 tablespoon olive oil in a skillet and cook 10 cherry tomatoes over high heat for 2 minutes. Add 1¾ cups tomato puree or tomato sauce and 2 tablespoons sun-dried tomato paste, bring to a boil, and cook for 2 minutes. Add the ravioli and toss well. Serve sprinkled with grated Parmesan.

Spinach and Ricotta Cannelloni with Tomato Sauce

Place 1 (12 oz) package washed spinach leaves in a saucepan with 1 tablespoon cold water and cook over medium heat, stirring occasionally, until wilted. Remove from the heat, transfer to a colander, and squeeze out as much water as possible, then place in a mixing bowl with 1 cup ricotta cheese and 1 teaspoon ground nutmeg. Mix well and season with black pepper. Take 4 large lasagna noodles and divide the ricotta and spinach mixture among them down the center lengthwise. Roll up the lasagna noodles to enclose the filling and place the "tubes" in a rectangular shallow gratin dish. Pour 1¼ cups prepared tomato sauce over the noodles and sprinkle with 2 tablespoons grated Parmesan cheese. Bake in a preheated oven, at 425°F, for 15 minutes, until piping hot. Serve with garlic bread and salad.

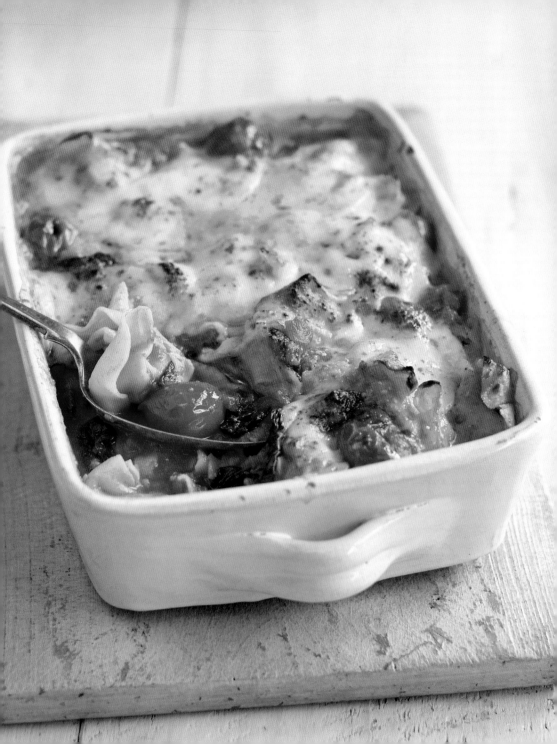

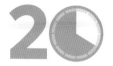

Chicken, Pesto, and Bacon Pan-Fry

Serves 4

4 (5 oz) chicken breasts
¼ cup pesto
4 good-quality bacon slices
2 tablespoons olive oil

To serve

seasonal vegetables
new potatoes (optional)

- Make a slit in each chicken breast along its length. Open and fill with the pesto. Stretch each bacon slice with the back of a sharp knife to lengthen, then wrap tightly around the chicken breast to enclose the pesto filling.

- Heat the oil in a large, heavy skillet and cook the chicken breasts over medium-high heat for 10–12 minutes, until golden and cooked through.

- Serve the chicken with seasonal vegetables and new potatoes, if desired.

Chicken, Bacon, and Pesto Stir-Fry

Heat 2 tablespoons olive oil in a wok or large, heavy skillet and cook 12 oz chicken breast strips over high heat for 3–4 minutes. Add 6 coarsely chopped bacon slices and cook for another 3 minutes, until golden. Add 10 halved cherry tomatoes and stir-fry for another 2 minutes, then add 2 tablespoons pesto and heat for 1 minute, until piping hot. Serve with warm crusty bread.

Chicken and Pesto Burgers With Bacon

Put 1 lb ground chicken in a food processor with 2 tablespoons pesto, season with black pepper, and process briefly to blend together. Shape the mixture, using hands lightly coated with flour (or cornmeal), into 4 patties and set aside. Heat 3 tablespoons olive oil in a large, heavy skillet and cook the burgers over high heat for 7–8 minutes on each side, until golden and cooked through. Meanwhile, cook 4 bacon slices under a preheated broiler for 4–5 minutes, until golden and cooked. Serve the burgers in whole-wheat buns with a spoonful of prepared white sauce or salsa on each and topped with a bacon slice. Top with arugula or the children's favourite salad leaves and serve.

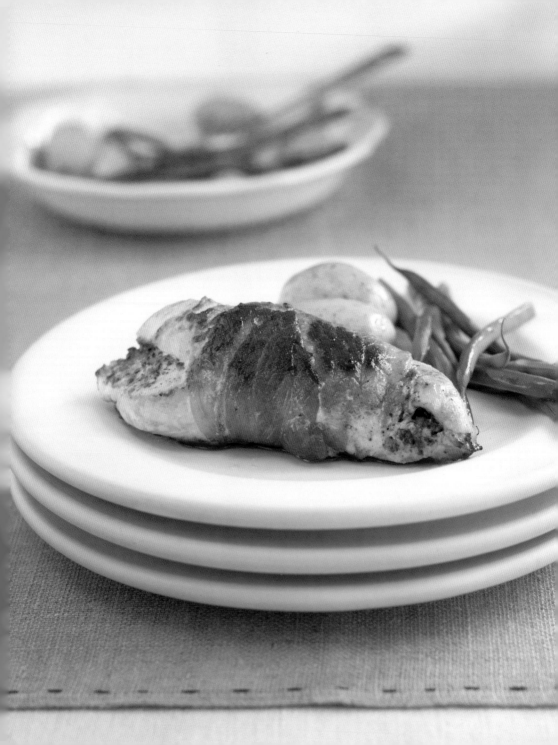

30 Spaghetti with Meat Sauce

Serves 4

8 oz spaghetti
2 tablespoons olive oil
1 onion, finely chopped
2 garlic cloves, crushed
1 large carrot, peeled and
  finely chopped
1 cup coarsely chopped
  mushrooms
1 teaspoon dried oregano
½ teaspoon dried thyme
12 oz ground round or
  ground sirloin beef
1¼ cups beef stock
1¼ cups tomato puree
  or tomato sauce
grated Parmesan cheese, to serve

- Bring a large saucepan of lightly salted water to a boil, cook the spaghetti according to the package directions, until tender, then drain and keep warm.

- Meanwhile, heat the oil in a large, heavy saucepan. Add the onion and cook over high heat for 2–3 minutes, then add the garlic, carrot, and mushrooms and cook for 5 minutes. Add the herbs and ground beef and cook for 10 minutes, until the meat is brown. Add the stock and tomato puree or sauce and continue to cook for another 10 minutes, stirring occasionally, until the sauce has thickened and the meat and vegetables are tender and cooked through.

- Add the spaghetti to the pan, mix with the meat and vegetables, and serve piled into warm serving bowls with the grated Parmesan on top.

 Meat Ravioli with Tomato Sauce

Cook 1 (11 oz) package meat ravioli in lightly salted boiling water according to package directions. Meanwhile, heat 2 tablespoons olive oil in a saucepan and cook 8 chopped tomatoes and 1 crushed clove garlic for 3 minutes, stirring continuously. Add 2 tablespoons tomato paste and ⅔ cup vegetable stock and bring to a boil. Transfer to a food processor and process until smooth. Toss into the drained pasta in a pan and stir. Serve in warmed bowls sprinkled with grated Parmesan cheese.

 Fusilli with Meat Sauce Gratin

Cook 1 lb fusilli pasta in a large saucepan of lightly salted boiling water according to the package directions, then drain and set aside. Meanwhile, heat a large skillet and cook 12 oz ground round or ground sirloin beef for 10 minutes, stirring occasionally, until well browned. Add 1¾ cups prepared tomato sauce and ⅓ cup chopped basil. Cover and simmer for 5 minutes. Add the drained pasta, transfer to a shallow gratin dish, and sprinkle with ⅓ cup grated Parmesan cheese. Cook under a preheated broiler for 2–3 minutes, until golden and bubbling, then serve with salad and garlic bread.

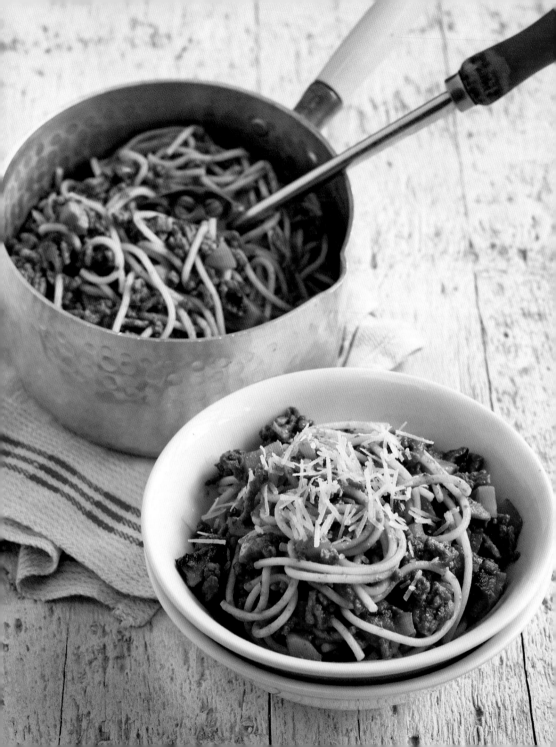

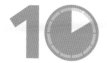

Frankfurter and Zucchini Frittata

Serves 4

2 tablespoons olive oil

1 large zucchini, cut into small chunks

6 frankfurters, chopped

6 eggs, beaten

⅔ cup crumbled feta cheese

black pepper

salad, to serve

- Heat the oil in a medium, nonstick skillet. Add the zucchini and frankfurters and cook, stirring, for 3 minutes, until the zucchini has softened.

- Season the eggs with black pepper (there is no need to add salt because the feta is salty). Pour into the skillet and cook, stirring gently, until the mixture starts to set. Sprinkle with the feta cheese.

- Place the skillet under a preheated hot broiler, keeping the handle away from the heat, and cook for 1 minute, until the top is set. Cut into wedges and serve with salad.

Frankfurter and Zucchini Omelet

Heat 2 tablespoons olive oil in a nonstick skillet, add 1 chopped onion and 1 chopped zucchini, and sauté, stirring occasionally, for 5 minutes, until the onion has softened and is starting to brown. Add 4 chopped frankfurters and cook for 2 minutes. Lightly beat 6 eggs and season with black pepper. Pour into the skillet and sprinkle with 4 halved cherry tomatoes and 1⅓ cups crumbled feta cheese. Cook the omelet, stirring lightly, until most of the egg has set. Carefully turn the omelet out of the skillet, then slide it back in to cook the other side. Serve cut into wedges with peas.

Simple Frankfurter and Zucchini

Quiche Cook 1 chopped zucchini in 2 tablespoons olive oil for 3 minutes, until softened and just starting to brown. Sprinkle over the bottom of a prepared pie crust with 4 chopped frankfurters and 1⅓ cups crumbled feta cheese. Mix together 4 beaten eggs and ⅔ cup light cream. Season lightly with black pepper and pour the filling into the pie crust. Bake in a preheated oven, at 400°F, for 20 minutes, until the filling has just set.

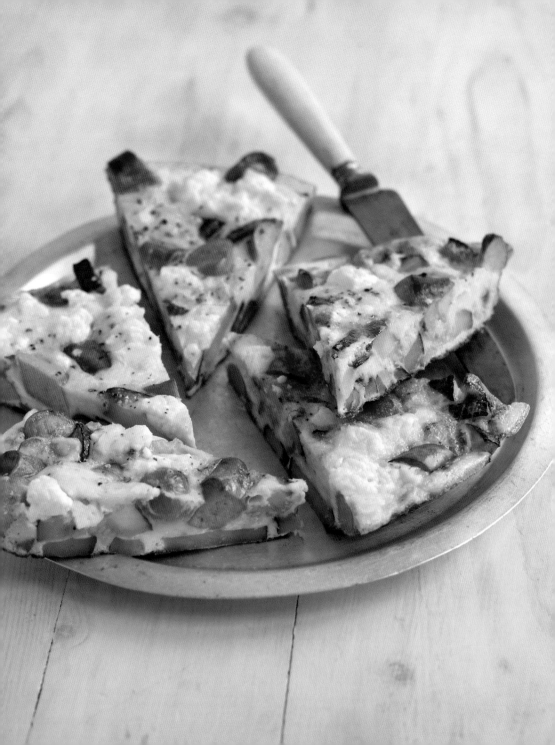

QuickCook

For All The Family

Recipes listed by cooking time

30

20

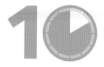

Curried Chicken, Mango, and Coconut Stir-Fry

Serves 4

1 tablespoon oil

12 oz boneless, skiness chicken
  strips, coarsely chopped

2 cups prepared fresh mango
  pieces, or 1 peeled, pitted,
  and diced managao

2 teaspoons curry powder

1 (1 lb) package mixed
  stir-fry vegetables

1 cup coconut milk

To serve

mango chutney (optional)

whole-wheat chapattis (optional)

- Heat the oil in a large, heavy skillet and cook the chicken over high heat for 4–5 minutes, until golden and cooked through. Add the mango and curry powder and stir-fry for another minute.

- Add the stir-fry vegetables and cook over high heat for 3 minutes, until the vegetables are just tender but still retaining their shape. Add the coconut milk and heat for 1 minute, until piping hot.

- Serve with mango chutney and whole-wheat chapattis, if desired.

 Coconuty Chicken and Mango Korma

Heat 1 tablespoon oil in a heavy skillet and cook 12 oz chicken breast pieces and 1 small finely chopped onion for 7–8 minutes, until brown. Add 2 tablespoons mild korma curry paste and cook for 1 minute. Add 1 mango, cut into chunks, and cook for 1 minute, stirring. Add 1¾ cups coconut milk and ⅔ cup chicken stock and bring to a boil. Reduce the heat and simmer for 5 minutes. Meanwhile, blend 2 teaspoons cornstarch with 2 tablespoons water. Add to the curry and stir until thick. Add ¼ cup chopped cilantro and serve with warm naan or rice.

 Chicken, Mango, and Coconut Biryani Cook 1 cup long-grain rice in a large saucepan of lightly salted boiling water according to the package directions, until tender, adding 1 cup frozen peas for the final 5 minutes of cooking. Heat 2 tablespoons oil in a large, heavy skillet and cook 8 oz coarsely chopped chicken breast strips and 1 sliced onion for 7–8 minutes, until brown and cooked through. Add 2 tablespoons mild curry paste and stir, then add 1¾ cups coconut milk and bring to a boil. Reduce the heat, cover, and simmer for 10 minutes, stirring occasionally, until the coconut

milk has reduced by half. For the final 2 minutes, add 2 cups prepared fresh mango pieces or 1 peeled, pitted, and diced mango. Drain the rice and peas, add to the skillet with ⅓ cup chopped cilantro, and toss well. Serve in warmed serving bowls.

KID-FORA-NUY

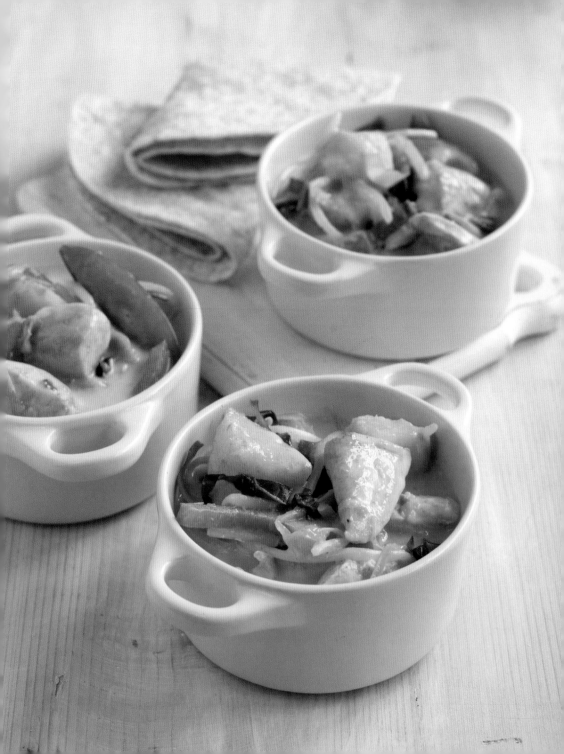

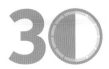

Cheesy Pesto Baked Potatoes

Serves 4

4 small/medium baking potatoes
4 cups spinach leaves
1 tablespoon water
2 tablespoons pesto
¼ cup grated Parmesan cheese
black pepper
baked beans, to serve

- Place the potatoes on a microwave-proof plate and pierce several times with a sharp knife, then cook for 5 minutes in a microwave. Turn and cook again for another 3 minutes, then transfer to the top of a preheated oven, at 425°F, for 5 minutes to make a little crisp.

- Meanwhile, place the spinach in a saucepan with the measured water and heat over medium heat for 5 minutes, until wilted.

- Remove the potatoes from the oven, cut in half lengthwise, and scoop out most of the flesh, reserving the skins. Put the potato flesh into a bowl and season with black pepper. Mash and stir with the pesto, then fold in the spinach leaves.

- Place the potato halves on a baking sheet, pile the pesto potato flesh back into the skins, and sprinkle with the Parmesan. Cook under a preheated broiler for 5 minutes, until golden and bubbling. Serve with baked beans.

 Cheesy Pesto Mashed Potatoes

Mix 2½ cups chilled prepared mashed potato with 2 tablespoons pesto, 3 tablespoons grated Parmesan cheese, and 1 egg. Heat 1 tablespoon butter in a nonstick skillet, press the potato mixture into the bottom, and cook over medium heat for 4 minutes. Sprinkle with 2 tablespoons grated Parmesan and place the skillet under a preheated broiler (keeping the handle away from the heat) and cook for 2 minutes, until golden. Serve in wedges.

 Cheesy Potato and Pesto Hash

Microwave ½ (26 oz) package of potato wedges with herbs according to package directions, until tender. Heat 3 tablespoons vegetable oil in a nonstick skillet and cook 1 chopped onion for 2 minutes. Coarsely chop the cooked potatoes, add to the onion, and cook for 5 minutes, stirring occasionally, until brown and crisp in places. Add 2 tablespoons pesto, stir, and cook for another 2–3 minutes. Remove from the heat and sprinkle with ¼ cup grated Parmesan cheese. Place the skillet under a preheated broiler (keeping the handle away from the heat) and cook for 2–3 minutes, until golden and bubbling. Serve hot.

KID-FORA-FUN

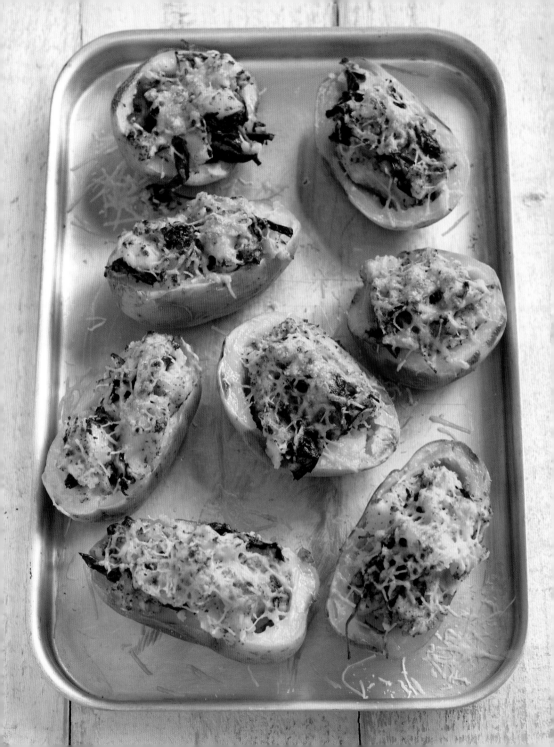

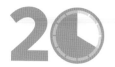

Hash Browns with Bacon and Mushrooms

Serves 4

4 russet or Yukon gold potatoes, peeled and shredded

1 parsnip, peeled and shredded

2 tablespoons butter

2 tablespoons sunflower oil

8 bacon slices

2 cups cremini mushrooms, halved, if large

salt and black pepper

To serve

baked beans

ketchup

- Squeeze out any moisture from the shredded potatoes and parsnips. Mix together in a bowl and season with salt and black pepper. Heat the butter and 1 tablespoon of the oil in a large, nonstick skillet. When the butter is melted and foaming, add the potato mixture and spread out evenly. Cook over medium heat for about 5 minutes, until the bottom is golden and crisp.

- Place a large plate or baking sheet over the skillet and turn the potato cake out. Slide it back into the skillet and cook for about 10 minutes, until the potato and parsnip are tender and golden.

- Meanwhile, heat the remaining oil in a separate skillet. Add the bacon and mushrooms and cook for 5 minutes, until the bacon is crisp and the mushrooms are tender.

- Cut the potato cake into wedges and serve with the bacon, mushrooms, baked beans, and ketchup.

Bacon and Mushroom Hash

Drain 1 (14½ oz) can new potatoes and cut into quarters. Cook in a large skillet with 2 tablespoons sunflower oil, 4 chopped bacon slices, and 2 cups halved mushrooms for 5 minutes, until golden. Add a sprinkle of Cajun seasoning and a handful of frozen peas. Cook, stirring, for a few minutes, until the peas are hot. Serve with sour cream and crusty bread.

Bacon and Cabbage Potato

Cake Cook 4 peeled and chopped russet potatoes in lightly salted boiling water for 10 minutes, until tender. Drain and mash with 2 tablespoons butter, a dash of milk, and salt and black pepper. Cook 1 (12 oz) package mixed frozen vegetables, drain, and coarsely mash. (Or use any leftover mashed potatoes and vegetables you may have.) Stir the vegetables into the potatoes. Cook 4 chopped bacon slices in a large nonstick skillet for 3 minutes, until crisp. Remove the bacon from the skille and stir into the potato mixture. Add 2 tablespoons sunflower oil to the bacon fat in the skillet and heat. Spoon in the potato mixture and spread evenly. Cook for 5 minutes, until golden and crisp underneath, then turn over and cook for another 5–10 minutes. Serve in wedges topped with fried eggs.

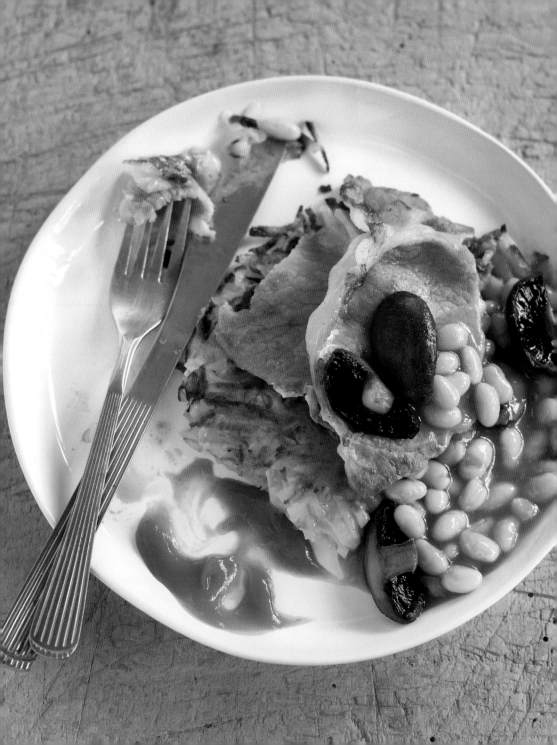

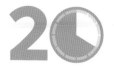

Hearty Bean, Bacon, and Pasta Soup

Serves 4

2 tablespoons olive oil

4 oz bacon, coarsely chopped

1 small onion, coarsely chopped

1 celery stick

1 carrot, peeled and coarsely chopped

4 cups rinsed and drained, canned mixed beans, such as kidney beans, great Northern beans, and chickpeas

2 tablespoons tomato paste

2½ cups chicken stock

4 oz pasta shapes

To serve

grated Parmesan cheese

chopped parsley, (optional)

warm crusty bread

- Heat the oil in a large, heavy saucepan and cook the bacon, onion, celery, and carrot for 5 minutes. Add the beans, tomato paste, and stock and bring to a boil. Reduce the heat and simmer for 10 minutes.

- Cook the pasta shapes in a small saucepan of lightly salted boiling water according to the package directions, until tender. Drain and set aside.

- Place the bean and stock mixture in a food processor and process until smooth. Return to the pan, add the pasta, and heat for 1 minute. Ladle into serving bowls and sprinkle with Parmesan and parsley, if desired. Serve with warm crusty bread.

---

10 Quick Bean Soup with Crispy Bacon

Place 2 cups canned, rinsed and drained, mixed beans, such as kidney beans, great Northern beans, and chickpeas, into a food processor with 1 (14½ oz) can diced tomatoes and process until smooth. Transfer to a large, heavy saucepan with 2 tablespoons tomato paste and 1¼ cups chicken stock and bring to a boil. Season well and ladle into soup bowls. Serve sprinkled with 1 tablespoon prepared croutons and crispy bacon bits.

30 Bean and Bacon Pasta Gratin

Heat 2 tablespoons olive oil in a large skillet and cook 4 oz coarsely chopped bacon, 1 small coarsely chopped onion, 1 celery stick, and 1 peeled and coarsely chopped carrot over medium heat for 5 minutes, until softened. Add 2 cups rinsed and drained, canned mixed beans, such as kidney beans, great Northern beans, and chickpeas, 1 (14½ oz) can diced tomatoes, and 1 tablespoon tomato paste. Bring to a boil, stirring, then remove from the heat. Meanwhile, cook 8 oz pasta shells in a large saucepan of lightly salted boiling water according to package directions, until tender. Drain, add to the bacon and beans, stir, and toss well. Transfer to a large gratin dish, sprinkle with 1 cup shredded cheddar cheese and, cook under a preheated hot broiler for 5 minutes, until golden and bubbling. Serve hot with crusty bread and salad.

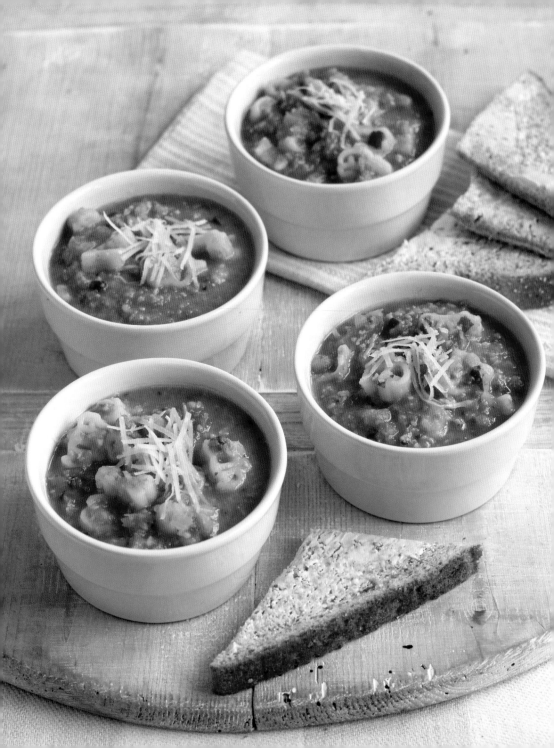

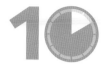

Kedgeree-Style Rice with Spinach

Serves 4

8 oz smoked haddock fillets

¾ cup frozen peas

⅔ cup boiling water

1 (10 oz) package spinach, thawed if frozen

2½ cups instant rice

2 tablespoons butter

½ teaspoon garam masala

bell pepper

3 tablespoons chopped parsley, to garnish (optional)

- Place the haddock and peas in a skillet, cover with the measured water, and bring to a boil. Reduce the heat, cover, and simmer for 3–4 minutes, adding the spinach for the final minute of cooking.

- Meanwhile, prepare the instant rice according to the package directions. Drain the fish, spinach, and peas and flake the fish. Return to the skillet and add the butter, garam masala, and rice, season with black pepper, and toss well.

- Serve sprinkled with parsley, if desired.

 Classic Kedgeree with Spinach

Cook 1¼ cups instant long-grain rice and 4 eggs in a saucepan of lightly salted boiling water according to the package directions, until the rice is tender, adding ¾ cup peas for the final few minutes. Meanwhile, place 8 oz smoked haddock or cod fillets in a skillet, pour about ⅔ cup water over the fish, cover with a tight-fitting lid, and bring to a boil. Cook for 5 minutes, until the fish is opaque and cooked through. Meanwhile, heat 2 tablespoons oil in a large, heavy skillet and cook 1 chopped onion over medium heat for 3–4 minutes. Add 2 tablespoons garam masala and cook for 1 minute, stirring, then add 1 (6 oz) package spinach leaves, toss, and cook

for 2–3 minutes, until the spinach has wilted. Drain the rice, removing the eggs. Add the rice and peas to the onion mixture and toss over the heat. Drain and flake the fish, add to the rice, and toss well. Shell the eggs and coarsely chop, then add to the rice and toss again. Serve on warmed serving plates.

Creamy Haddock and Spinach Risotto Heat 2 tablespoons olive oil in a saucepan and cook 1 chopped onion for 3–4 minutes, then add 1¼ cups risotto rice and 1 teaspoon garam masala and stir to coat in oil. Pour in 2½ cups fish stock, bring to a boil, reduce the heat, and simmer for 10 minutes, until the stock is absorbed. Add 2 cups fish stock, cover, and simmer for 2 minutes. Stir in 8 oz coarsely chopped smoked haddock fillets, ¾ cup frozen peas, and 1 (6 oz) package spinach. Increase the heat and cook for 5 minutes, until the fish is opaque and cooked. Season with black pepper, stir in 1 cup crème fraîche or light cream, and heat for 2–3 minutes, stirring until hot. Serve with crusty bread.

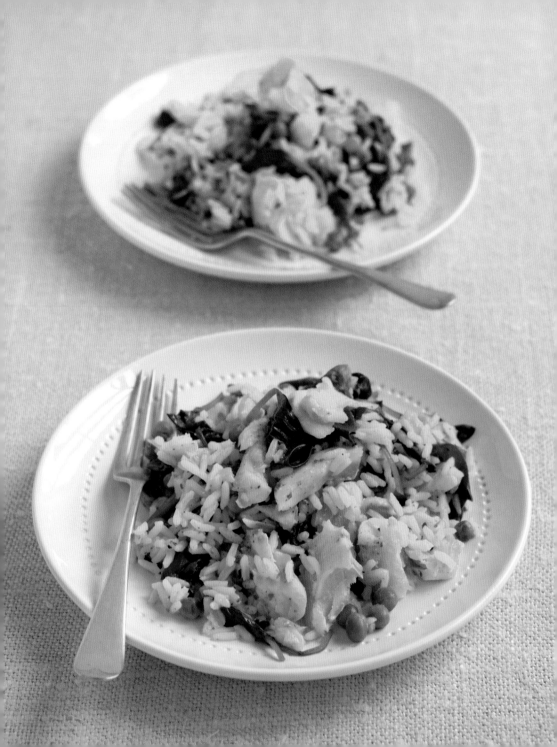

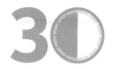

Warm Mozzarella, Chicken, Tomato, and Basil Pasta

Serves 4

8 oz penne
¼ tablespoons olive oil
8 oz skinless, boneless chicken breast, cut into strips
¼ cup pine nuts
8 cherry tomatoes, halved
⅓ cup chopped basil leaves
4 oz baby mozzarella balls, drained
black pepper

- Cook the penne in a large saucepan of lightly salted boiling water according to package directions, until tender. Drain and keep warm.

- Meanwhile, heat the oil in a large, heavy skillet and cook the chicken over high heat for 8–10 minutes, until golden and cooked through. Add the pine nuts and cook for another 2 minutes, until golden. Add the cherry tomato halves and toss and cook for another 2 minutes.

- Add the drained pasta to the pan and toss well, then stir in the chopped basil and season well with black pepper.

- Turn into a serving bowl and stir in the mozzarella balls.

Cheese-Filled Pasta with Tomatoes and Basil Cook 1 (11 oz) package 3-cheese-filled pasta in a saucepan of lightly salted boiling water according to package directions. Meanwhile, heat 3 tablespoons olive oil in a skillet and cook ¼ cup pine nuts for 1 minute, then add 10 halved cherry tomatoes and cook for 2–3 minutes, until softened but retaining their shape. Drain the pasta, toss into the pan with the tomatoes and pine nuts, and stir well. Transfer to warmed serving bowls and sprinkle with basil leaves.

Cheesy Tomato and Basil Pasta Melt Cook 8 oz pasta shapes in a large saucepan of lightly salted boiling water for 10 minutes, until tender. Drain and keep warm. Heat 1 tablespoon olive oil in a large skillet and cook ¼ cup pine nuts for 1 minute, then add 2½ cups whole cherry tomatoes over high heat for 2–3 minutes, until the tomatoes have softened. Add the drained pasta to the pan and toss well, then add ½ cup chopped basil leaves and season well with black pepper. Arrange in a medium gratin dish, then top with 10 oz sliced mozzarella cheese. Cook under a preheated medium broiler for 3–4 minutes, until golden and bubbling.

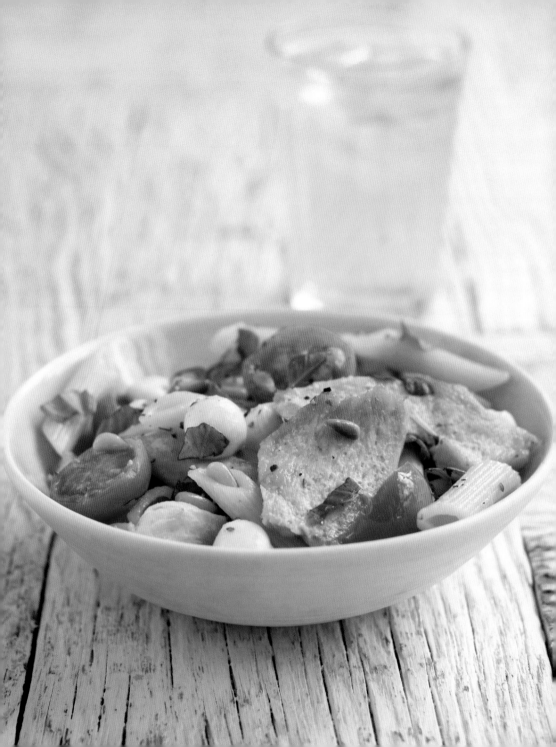

3⓿ Creamy Pork and Apple Pies

Serves 4

8 russet or Yukon gold potatoes,
  peeled and chopped
1 tablespoon sunflower oil
1 onion, chopped
1 lb boneless pork cutlets,
  cut into bite-size pieces
1 Pippin apple, peeled, cored,
  and chopped
2 cups sliced mushrooms
1 cup crème fraîche or light cream
½ cup chicken stock
1 teaspoon Dijon mustard
2 tablespoons butter
¼ cup milk
½ cup shredded cheddar cheese
salt and black pepper
peas, to serve
cherry tomatoes, basil leaves
and chives, to garnish

- Cook the potatoes in a large saucepan of lightly salted boiling water for 10–15 minutes, until tender.

- Meanwhile, heat the oil in a skillet. Add the onion and pork and cook over high heat for 5 minutes, stirring occasionally. Add the apple and mushrooms and cook for another 2 minutes. Stir in the crème fraîche or light cream, stock, and mustard and season with salt and black pepper. Simmer for 5 minutes.

- When the potatoes are cooked, drain and mash with the butter and milk and season with salt and black pepper. Spoon the pork mixture into individual flameproof dishes and spoon the mashed potatoes over the top. Make ridges in the potatoes with the back of a fork and sprinkle the cheese over the top. Cook under a preheated medium broiler until the cheese melts.

- Garnish the pies with animal faces using cherry tomatoes for noses, peas for eyes, basil leaves for ears, and chives for whiskers. Serve with peas.

1⓿ Creamy Pork and Apple

Cook 1 loaf prepared garlic bread in a preheated oven, at 450°F, for 10 minutes. Meanwhile, cook 4 thin (4 oz) pork cutlets for 3 minutes, turning once. Add 1 sliced apple, cook for 1 minute, then stir in 1½ cups prepared mushroom pasta sauce. Bring to a boil and simmer for 5 minutes. Serve with the garlic bread.

2⓿ Curried Pork and Apple Phyllo Pies

Cut 1 lb pork cutlets into small chunks and cook in 1 tablespoon sunflower oil for 5 minutes, until browned and just cooked. Stir in 2 tablespoons mild curry paste, cook for 1 minute, then add 1¾ cups coconut milk. Bring to a boil, reduce the heat, and simmer for 5 minutes. Stir in 1 chopped Pippin apple, ⅓ cup golden raisins, and

2 tablespoons chopped cilantro. Brush 4 sheets of phyllo pastry with 4 tablespoons butter, melted, and ruffle to make 4 scrunched circles to fit the tops of 4 individual pie dishes. Spoon the curry into dishes. Place the phyllo on top, sprinkle with sesame seeds, and bake in a preheated oven, at 450°F, for 10 minutes, until the pastry is golden. Serve with green beans.

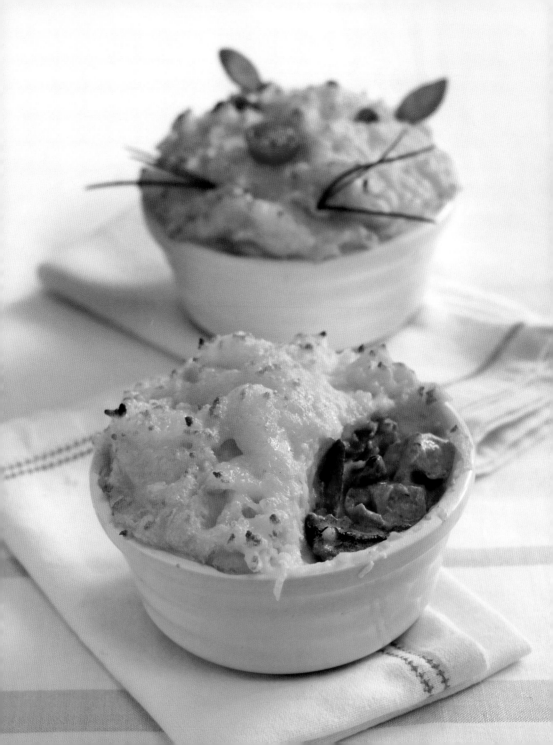

30 Spiced Rice and Chickpea Balls with Sweet Chili sauce

Serves 4

½ cup risotto rice
1¼ cups vegetable stock
1 teaspoon minced garlic
1 teaspoon ground cumin
1 teaspoon ground coriander
½ teaspoon paprika
¼ teaspoon turmeric
3 tablespoons chopped cilantro
1 (15 oz) can chickpeas,
  rinsed and drained
1 egg yolk
1 cup cornmeal
⅓ cup sesame seeds
¼ cup vegetable oil
black pepper
sweet chili sauce, to serve

- Place the rice in a small saucepan with the stock and bring to a boil. Reduce the heat, cover, and simmer according to the package directions, until the rice is tender and sticky. Stir in the garlic, spices, and chopped cilantro.

- Meanwhile, put the chickpeas in a food processor and process until almost smooth but still retaining some texture. Add the cooked sticky rice to the bowl with the egg yolk and process together, then season with black pepper.

- Mix together the cornmeal and sesame seeds in a bowl. Form the chickpea mixture into walnut-size balls and coat in the cornmeal mixture. Heat the oil in a large, heavy skillet and cook over high heat for 4–5 minutes, turning occasionally, until crisp and golden.

- Drain on paper towels and serve with sweet chili sauce for dipping.

10 Spiced Chickpea Puree and Sweet Chili Pita Breads

Place 1 (15 oz) can chickpeas, rinsed and drained, in a saucepan with the juice and bring to a boil. Reduce the heat and simmer for 4 minutes, until piping hot. Drain and transfer to a food processor with 1 tablespoon olive oil, ½ teaspoon each of ground cumin, ground coriander, and paprika, and 3 tablespoons chopped cilantro. Squeeze in the juice of 1 lemon and process until smooth. Lightly toast 4 mini pita breads, then split and fill with the puree along with a handful of spinach leaves and a drizzle of sweet chili sauce.

20 Spicy Chickpea Cakes with Sweet Chili sauce

Process 1 (15 oz) can chickpeas, drained and rinsed, in a food processor with 1 teaspoon minced garlic, ½ teaspoon each of ground cumin, coriander, and paprika, ¼ teaspoon turmeric, ¾ cup dry whole-wheat bread crumbs, and 1 egg yolk. Divide into 4 patties. Heat 3 tablespoons vegetable oil in a large, heavy skillet and cook the patties for 2 minutes on each side. Serve with sweet chili sauce.

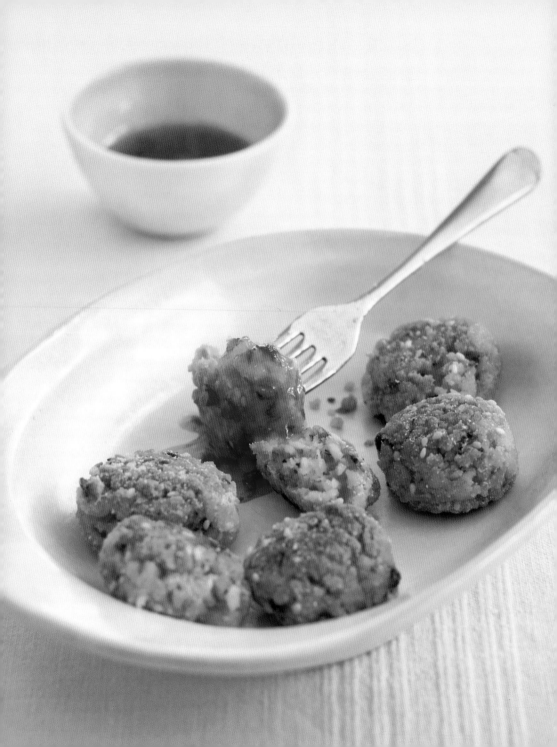

3⦿ Chile and Mustard Turkey Meatballs and Herb Tomato Sauce

Serves 4

12 oz ground turkey
¼ cup chopped parsley
½ classic red chile, seeded and
  finely chopped
1 tablespoon whole-grain mustard
all-purpose flour, for dusting
3 tablespoons olive oil
2 cups tomato puree
  or tomato sauce
¼ cup chopped basil
8 oz spaghetti
grated Parmesan cheese, to serve
  (optional)

- Place the ground turkey in a food processor with the parsley, chile, and mustard and process until well blended. Remove from the bowl and, using well-floured hands, shape the mixture into about 12–16 small walnut-size balls.

- Heat the oil in a large, heavy skillet and cook the meatballs over medium heat for 10–15 minutes, turning frequently, until the balls are golden and cooked through. Add the tomato puree or tomato sauce and basil and cook for another 5 minutes, until piping hot.

- Cook the spaghetti in a large saucepan of lightly salted boiling water according to the package directions, until tender. Drain and keep warm.

- Serve the meatballs and tomato sauce on top of the spaghetti in warmed serving bowls. Sprinkle with Parmesan, if desired.

 1⦿ Spicy Turkey Strips in a Tomato and Mustard Sauce Slice 12 oz turkey cutlets into thin strips. Heat 3 tablespoons vegetable oil in a large skillet and cook the turkey for 5 minutes, until golden, stirring occasionally. Add 1 teaspoon mild chili powder and stir to coat. Add 1¼ cups tomato puree or tomato sauce and some black pepper and bring to a boil. Cover and simmer for 3 minutes. Add 1 tablespoon whole-grain mustard and 1 tablespoon chopped parsley and serve with rice or mashed potatoes.

 2⦿ Chile and Mustard Turkey Burgers and Homemade Tomato Sauce Place 12 oz ground turkey in a food processor with ¼ cup chopped parsley, ½ seeded and finely chopped classic red chile, and 1 tablespoon whole-grain mustard and process until well blended. Divide the mixture into 4 portions, then shape into patties. Heat 1 tablespoon olive oil in a large, heavy nonstick skillet and cook the patties over medium heat for 3–4 minutes on each side, until golden and cooked through. Meanwhile, make the tomato sauce. Place ⅔ cup tomato puree or tomato sauce in a small saucepan with 1 tablespoon red wine vinegar, 2 tablespoons light brown sugar, and ½ teaspoon paprika. Begin to heat, stirring continually, increasing the heat but being careful the tomato puree does not spit while cooking, until the sugar has melted and the sauce is smooth. Transfer to a small serving bowl. Put the burgers into sliced whole-wheat burger buns, spoon the tomato sauce over them, and serve with salad.

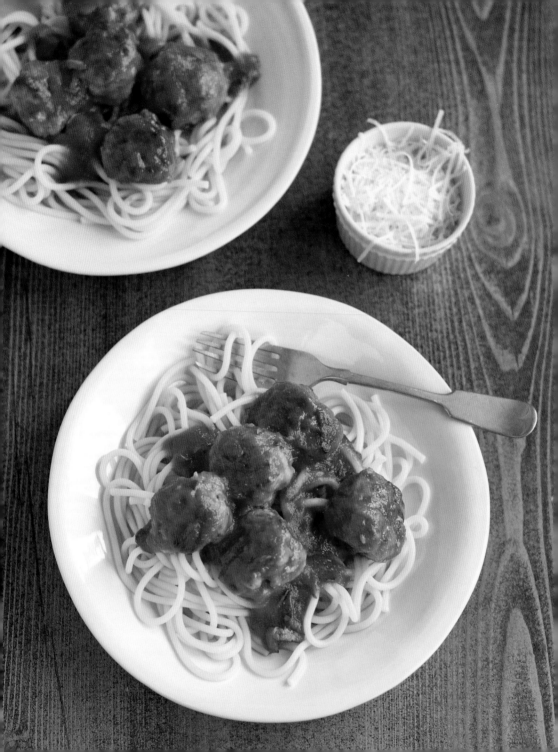

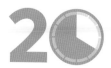

Gnocchi Pasta Gratin

Serves 4

1 (1 lb) package gnocchi

2 tablespoons olive oil

1½ cups prepared arrabbiata tomato sauce

¼ cup sun-dried tomato paste

1¼ cups pitted ripe black olives, drained

5 oz mozzarella cheese, drained and thinly sliced

¼ cup grated pecorino cheese

bell pepper

basil leaves, to garnish

To serve

garlic bread (optional)

salad (optional)

- Cook the gnocchi in a large saucepan of lightly salted boiling water according to the package directions, then drain. Toss with the oil and season with bell pepper.

- Meanwhile, place the arrabbiata sauce and sun-dried tomato paste in a saucepan and heat for 2 minutes, until hot. Toss the gnocchi into the sauce and add the olives. Toss well, then transfer to a shallow gratin dish and arrange the mozzarella slices on top. Sprinkle the grated pecorino over the top of the mozzarella, then cook under a preheated hot broiler for 8–10 minutes, until golden and bubbling.

- Serve hot, garnished with basil leaves, with garlic bread and salad, if desired.

10 Gnocchi with Cherry Tomato

Sauce Cook the gnocchi in a large saucepan of lightly salted boiling water according to the package directions, then drain and return to the pan. Add 1 tablespoon olive oil and season with black pepper. Add 1¾ cups cherry tomato sauce from a jar and 2 tablespoons sun-dried tomato paste and cook over medium heat for 5 minutes, until piping hot and cooked through. Serve in warmed serving bowls with grated pecorino.

30 Creamy Gnocchi and Eggplant

Casserole Cook 1 (1 lb) package gnocchi in a large saucepan of lightly salted boiling water according to the package directions. Meanwhile, heat 2 cups prepared tomato sauce for 2–3 minutes, until piping hot. Drain the gnocchi well and toss with 1 (12 oz) jar roasted peppers, drained, 1 (10½ oz) jar eggplant antipasti, and the hot tomato sauce. Transfer to a large gratin dish. Mix 1¼ cups plain yogurt with 2 eggs and 2 tablespoons grated Parmesan cheese. Pour over the top of the gnocchi and spread evenly to the edges. Sprinkle with 3 tablespoons grated Parmesan and bake in a preheated oven, at 425°F, for 20 minutes, until golden and piping hot.

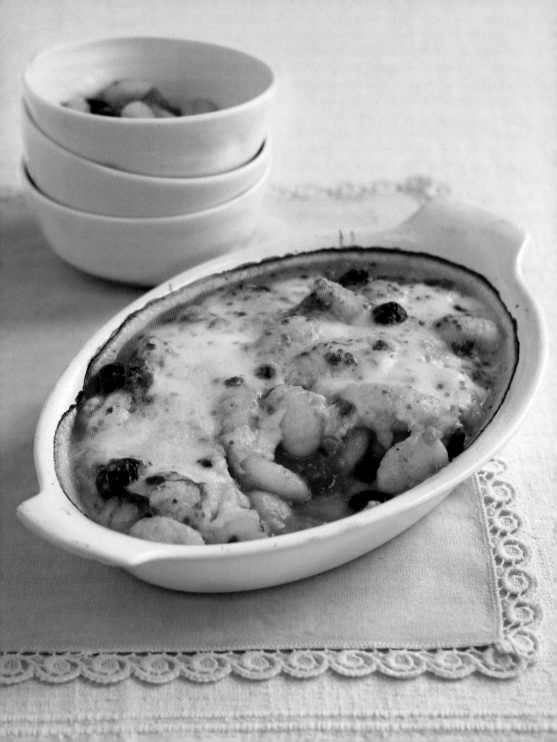

30 Tuna, Bell Pepper, and Cheese Calzones

Makes 4

1 (5 oz) package pizza crust mix
flour, for dusting
1 (5 oz) can chunk light tuna
in water, drained
1 small green bell pepper, cored,
seeded, and coarsely chopped
½ cup shredded cheddar cheese
salad, to serve (optional)

- Put the pizza crust mix in a bowl and make up with warm water according to the package directions. Divide into 4 portions, place on a lightly floured surface, and knead briefly to produce smooth balls of dough. Roll out each ball to about an 8 inch circle.

- Mix together the tuna, green bell pepper, and cheese in a bowl, then divide the mixture among the 4 circles. Lightly brush the rims with a little cold water, then fold the dough over the filling and press to form a semicircle. Place the 4 semicircles on baking sheets and bake in a preheated oven, at 425°F, for 15–18 minutes, until golden and cooked.

- Serve hot or warm with salad, if desired.

1 Tuna, Bell Pepper, and Cheese Wraps

Mix 1 (5 oz) can chunk light tuna in water, drained, with ½ cored, seeded, and thinly sliced green bell pepper and 1 tablespoon mayonnaise and season with black pepper. Spread the tuna mayonnaise over the top of 2 flour tortillas, sprinkle each with ¼ cup shredded cheddar cheese, and roll tightly to form a pinwheel effect. Cut each in half and serve with a handful of cherry tomato halves as a delicious dinner on the move.

2 Melted Tuna, Bell Pepper, and Cheese Triangles

Place 1 (5 oz) can chunk light tuna in water, drained, in a bowl with 1 small cored, seeded, and chopped green bell pepper, 1 small cored, seeded, and chopped red bell pepper, and ½ cup shredded cheddar cheese. Use to fill each of 4 flour tortillas in one-quarter of the circle. Fold the wraps into 4 to enclose the filling, then place in a shallow flameproof dish. Arrange 5 oz drained and thinly sliced mozzarella over the tortillas, sprinkle over another ¼ cup shredded cheddar cheese, and cook under a preheated broiler for 5 minutes, until hot, bubbling and golden. Serve with a simple salad.

KID-FORA-CAJ

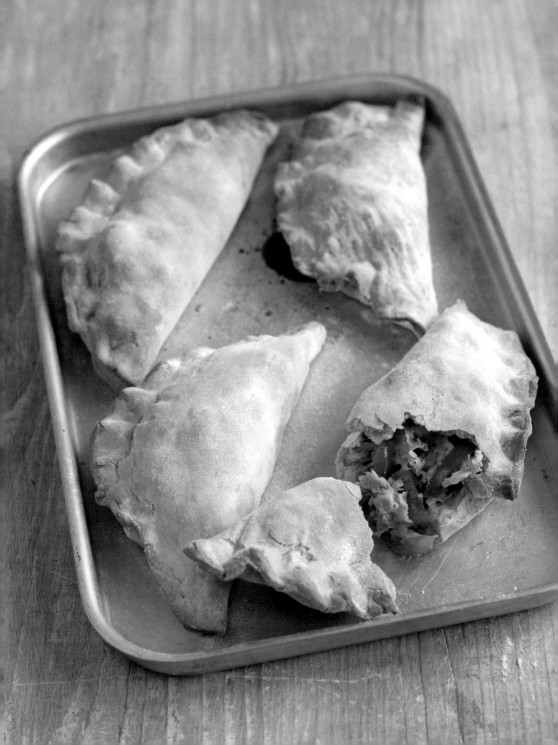

30 Scrambled Egg Enchiladas with Spinach and Tomatoes

Serves 4

3 tablespoons olive oil
1 small red onion, chopped
1 garlic clove, crushed
1 small red bell pepper, cored, seeded, and cut into strips
1 red chile, cored, seeded, and chopped
½ teaspoon smoked paprika
pinch of ground coriander
2 tablespoons butter
4 eggs, beaten
4 soft flour tortillas
2 handfuls of baby spinach leaves
¾ cup shredded cheddar cheese
2 tomatoes, chopped
salt and black pepper

- Heat the oil in a small skillet, add the onion, garlic, red bell pepper, and chile and cook over low heat, stirring occasionally, for 10 minutes, until soft and tender. Stir in the paprika and coriander, season with salt and black pepper, and cook for another 2 minutes.

- Melt the butter in a separate small saucepan (preferably nonstick). Season the eggs with salt and black pepper and pour into the pan. Cook over low heat, stirring, until the egg is softly set and scrambled, then remove from the heat.

- Lay the tortillas out on a board, arrange the spinach leaves on top, then spoon the onion mixture and the scrambled egg over the spinach. Fold the tortillas into triangles to enclose the filling and place in an ovenproof dish. Sprinkle the cheese and chopped tomatoes over the top and bake in a preheated oven, at 400°F, for 10 minutes, until the cheese is melted and bubbling.

 Scrambled Egg and Tomato Burritos

Beat 4 eggs and season with salt and black pepper, ½ teaspoon smoked paprika, and a pinch of ground cumin. Melt 2 tablespoons butter in a nonstick saucepan, add the eggs, and stir over low heat until softly scrambled. Spoon onto warmed soft tortillas with a spoonful of prepared tomato salsa and a handful of baby spinach leaves. Roll up to enclose the filling and serve.

 Mexican Baked Eggs

Heat 3 tablespoons olive oil in a skillet and sauté 1 chopped red onion, 1 crushed garlic clove, 2 cored, seeded, and sliced red bell peppers, and 1 seeded and chopped red bell pepper for 5 minutes to soften. Stir in ½ teaspoon smoked paprika, a pinch of ground cumin, and 2 chopped tomatoes. Season with salt and black pepper and cook for 5 minutes, stirring occasionally. Transfer to an ovenproof dish and make 4 dips in the mixture. Break an egg into each dip and sprinkle with ½ cup shredded cheddar cheese. Bake in a preheated oven, at 400°F, for 10 minutes, until the egg whites are set and the yolks still soft. Serve with warmed tortillas.

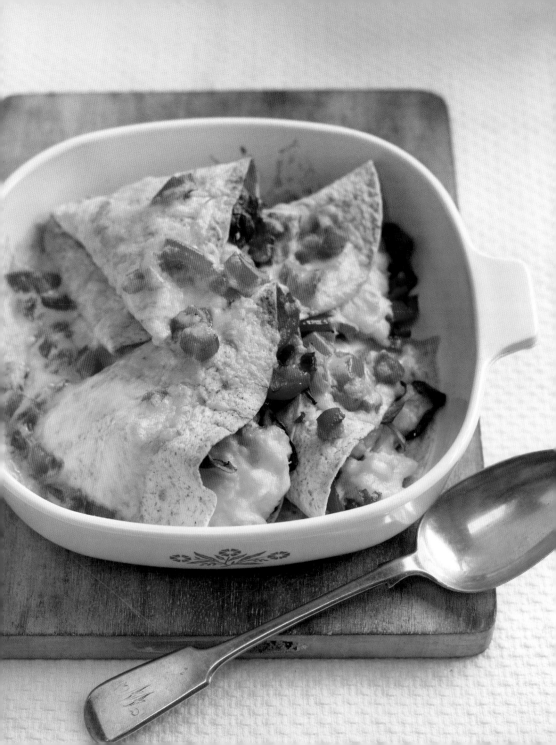

30 Beef Meatballs with Gravy and Baked Fries

Serves 4

2 baking potatoes, scrubbed
3 tablespoons sunflower oil
1 lb ground round or ground
  sirloin beef
½ onion, finely chopped
1 garlic clove, crushed
1 egg yolk
1 tablespoon all-purpose flour,
  plus extra for coating
1¼ cups rich beef stock
1 tablespoon tomato paste
salt and black pepper
broccoli, to serve

- Cut the potatoes into french-fry shapes and toss in 2 tablespoons of the oil. Spread over a baking sheet in a single layer and season with salt and black pepper. Bake in a preheated oven, at 425°F, for 25 minutes, turning occasionally, until golden and cooked through.

- Meanwhile, place the ground beef in a bowl with the onion, garlic, and egg yolk. Season with salt and black pepper and mix well. Roll the mixture into 12 even-size balls and roll in flour to coat. Heat the remaining oil in a large skillet, add the meatballs, and cook over medium heat for 10 minutes, turning occasionally, until browned and cooked through. Remove from the skillet and set aside.

- Add the flour to the skillet and cook, stirring, for 1 minute. Pour in the stock, bring to a boil, stir in the tomato paste, and simmer for 2 minutes. Remove from the heat and return the meatballs to the skillet and heat through. Serve with broccoli.

---

1 Spicy Tomato Meatballs with

Couscous Place 1½ cups couscous in a heatproof bowl and add enough boiling water to cover by ½ inch. Cover with plastic wrap and let stand for 5 minutes. Put 12 oz cooked Swedish-style meatballs into a saucepan, add 1½ cups prepared tomato sauce and a pinch of chili powder, and heat for 5 minutes. Add a pat of butter to the couscous, season, and fluff up with a fork until the butter has melted. Serve with the meatballs and tomato sauce.

2 Creamy Meatball Pasta

Cook 12 oz penne or rigatoni in a large saucepan of lightly salted boiling water according to the package directions, until just tender. Meanwhile, heat 2 tablespoons sunflower oil in a large skillet, add 12 oz prepared beef meatballs, and cook for 5 minutes, until browned and cooked through. Remove from the skillet and set aside. Add 2 cups sliced mushrooms and 1 chopped zucchini to the skillet and sauté for 2 minutes. Stir in ¼ cup crème fraîche or light cream and heat through, adding a little water if the sauce is too thick. Return the meatballs to the skillet and heat through. Drain the pasta, add to the skillet, and mix well. Add 2 tablespoons chopped parsley and sprinkle with grated cheese to serve.

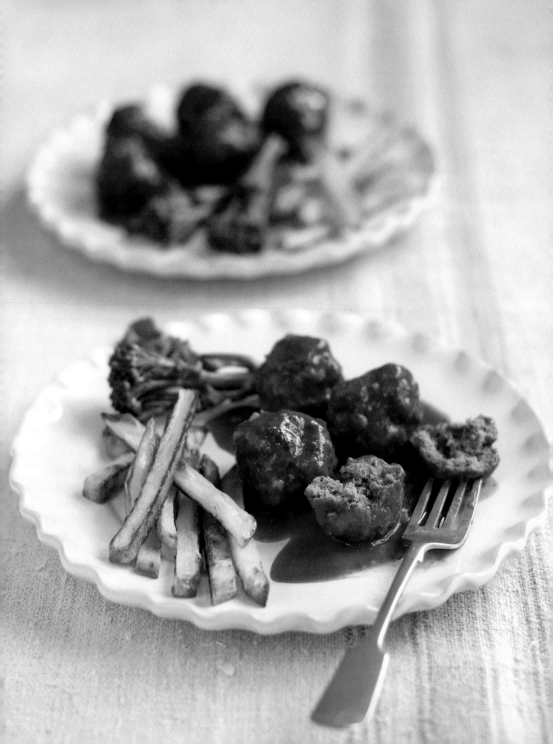

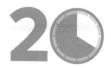

Salmon and Broccoli Fish Cakes

Makes 4

1 cup broccoli florets
¼ cup instant mashed potatoes
1 tablespoon grated Parmesan
 cheese
8 oz salmon fillet
¼ cup all-purpose flour,
 plus extra for dusting
1 egg, beaten
1½ cups dry whole-wheat
 bread crumbs
⅓ cup vegetable oil
mixed peas and corn, to serve
 (optional)

- Cook the broccoli in a saucepan of lightly salted boiling water for 3 minutes. Drain, rinse with cold water, and chop into small pieces. Make up the instant mashed potatoes according to the package directions, add the Parmesan, and mix well.

- Place the salmon on a microwave-proof plate and cover with plastic wrap. Cook for 2–3 minutes, until the fish is opaque.

- Mix the potato with the broccoli and salmon, then divide into 4 portions. Shape into patties, using metal spoons if the mixture is too hot to handle. Put the flour on one plate, the beaten egg on another, and the bread crumbs on a third. Lightly roll the fish cakes in the flour, then the egg, and finally the bread crumbs.

- Heat the oil in a large, heavy skillet and cook the fish cakes for 2–3 minutes on each side. Drain on paper towels and serve with peas and corn, if desired.

Pan-Fried Salmon and Broccoli

Season 2 (5 oz) salmon fillets with black pepper. Heat 1 tablespoon butter in a skillet and cook the fish for 5–7 minutes, turning once, until golden. Meanwhile, heat 2 tablespoons olive oil in a skillet and cook 3 cups broccoli florets for 5 minutes, turning occasionally and adding 2 tablespoons water for the final 2 minutes. Serve the salmon and broccoli with grated Parmesan cheese.

Salmon and Broccoli Pie

Cook 3 cups broccoli florets in lightly salted boiling water for 5 minutes, until just tender, then drain. Meanwhile, place 12 oz salmon fillets in a skillet with ⅔ cup water and bring to a boil, cover tightly, and simmer for 5 minutes, until the fish is opaque. Reserve the cooking liquid. Heat 2 tablespoons butter in a saucepan until melted. Add 2 tablespoons flour and cook over low heat for a few seconds. Remove from the heat and gradually add 1¼ cups milk,

a little at a time, stirring well. Once all the milk is added, return to the heat and bring to a boil, stirring until thickened. Stir in the reserved cooking liquid and ¼ cup grated Parmesan cheese. Flake the salmon, add to the sauce with the broccoli, and fold in. Transfer to a shallow gratin dish. Mix 4 cups chilled prepared mashed potato to loosen. Spoon it over the salmon and sprinkle with 3 tablespoons grated Parmesan. Cook under a preheated broiler for 5–8 minutes, until golden.

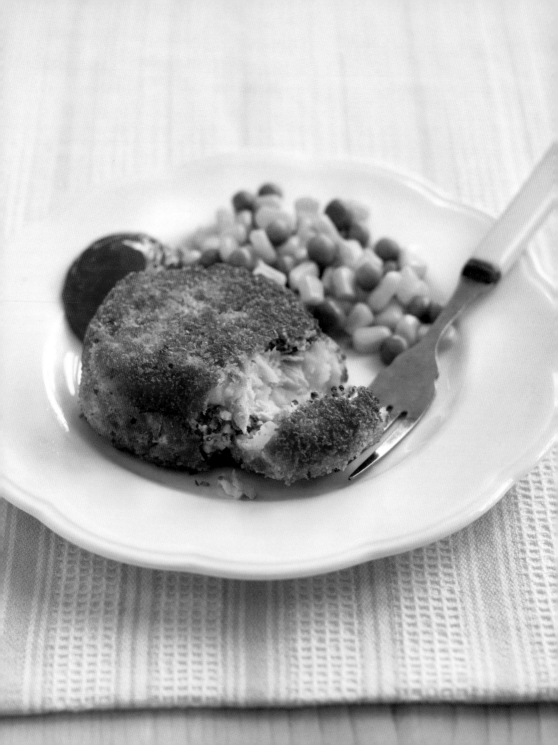

10 Creamy Pork and Roasted Peppers

Serves 4

2 tablespoons olive oil

12 oz pork tenderloin, cut into strips

1 tablespoon smoked paprika

1¼ cups prepared tomato sauce

⅔ cup sour cream

1 (12 oz) jar roasted peppers, drained

chopped parsley, to garnish

- Heat the oil in a large, heavy skillet and cook the pork over high heat for 5 minutes, until golden and cooked through.

- Add the paprika and cook for a few seconds, then add the tomato sauce and bring to a boil.

- Reduce the heat, add the sour cream and roasted peppers, and heat for 2–3 minutes, until piping hot but not boiling.

- Sprinkle with chopped parsley to serve, if desired.

 Creamy Pork Raxo

Heat 1 tablespoon olive oil in a large, heavy skillet and cook 1 small sliced red onion and 3 thinly sliced (5 oz) pork cutlets for 5 minutes, until browned. Add 2 teaspoons smoked paprika and ½ teaspoon ground cumin and cook for 1 minute, then add 2 tablespoons sun-dried tomato paste and ¾ cup canned diced tomatoes. Cook, stirring, for another 2 minutes, then add ⅓ cup water. Add 1 cup crème fraîche or light cream and cook, stirring, for another 2 minutes, until piping hot. Serve with rice or fries.

 Pork and Bell Pepper Goulash

Heat 1 tablespoon olive oil in a large, heavy saucepan and cook 1 large red onion, 1 cored, seeded, and chopped green bell pepper, 1 cored, seeded, and chopped red bell pepper, and 4 thinly sliced (5 oz) pork cutlets over high heat for 8–10 minutes, until the pork is browned. Add 1 tablespoon smoked paprika and 1 teaspoon ground cumin and cook for 1 minute, then add 1 (14½ oz) can diced tomatoes, 2 cups chicken stock, and 1 tablespoon sun-dried tomato paste and bring to a boil. Cover and simmer for 15 minutes. Serve ladled over hot rice with spoonfuls of sour cream and garnished with parsley, if desired.

KID-FORA-NED

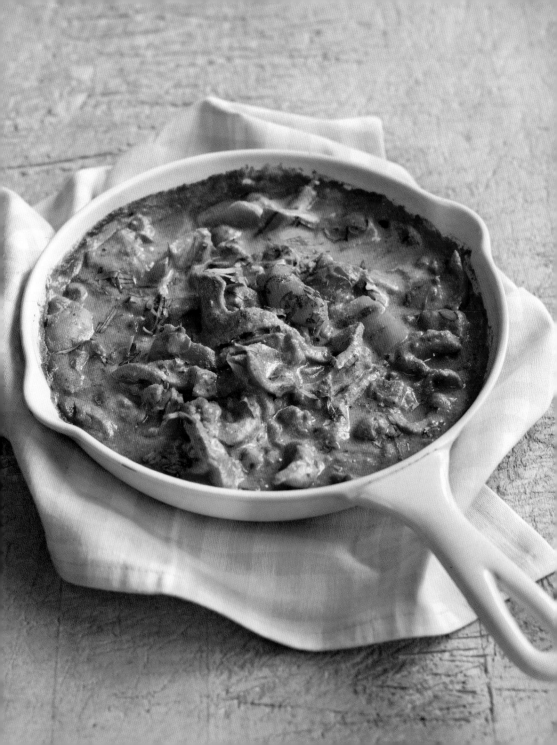

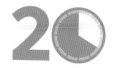

Lemon Cod Strips with Caperless Tartar Sauce

Serves 4

about 2½ cups vegetable oil
1 lb cod fillets, cut into chunky
  pieces
1 cup all-purpose flour
1 teaspoon paprika
2 eggs, beaten
2½ cups dry bread crumbs
3 tablespoons chopped parsley
grated rind of 1 lemon
black pepper
peas, to serve (optional)

For the tartar sauce

3 tablespoons mayonnaise
3 tablespoons crème fraîche
  or sour cream
½ teaspoon Dijon mustard
1 small pickle, finely chopped
1 tablespoon chopped parsley

- Pour the vegetable oil into a medium, deep saucepan and begin to heat, so it is ready to fry the fish.

- Meanwhile, place the cod pieces in a bowl, add the flour and paprika, and season with black pepper. Toss well to lightly coat the fish. Place the beaten eggs in one bowl, and mix the bread crumbs, parsley, and lemon rind in another. Toss the fish pieces in the egg, then in the lemon and herb bread crumbs, pressing firmly to coat.

- Test the oil to see if it is hot enough—lower a small piece of bread into the oil, and if it turns brown in 20 seconds, the oil is ready. Carefully lower the fish pieces into the hot oil and cook for 3–4 minutes, until browned and cooked through. Remove from the oil, using a slotted spoon, and drain on paper towels.

- To make the tartar sauce, mix the mayonnaise with the crème fraîche or sour cream and mustard, then fold in the chopped pickle and parsley.

- Serve the fish with the sauce to dip and peas, if desired.

Lemon and Paprika Cod Cubes with Herbed Mayonnaise Put 12 oz cubed cod in a bowl with 3 tablespoons all-purpose flour, ½ teaspoon paprika, and the grated rind of 1 lemon. Toss well. Heat ⅓ cup olive oil in a large, heavy skillet. Cook the fish cubes for 5 minutes, turning occasionally. Meanwhile, mix ⅓ cup mayonnaise with 1 tablespoon chopped herbs and serve with the fish.

Lemony Roasted Cod with Caperless Tartar Sauce Place 4 (4 oz) cod pieces in a lightly oiled, large roasting pan. Mix 8 oz halved baby new potatoes and 6 peeled and chunky cut carrots with 1 tablespoon olive oil and sprinkle around the fish. Sprinkle with 3 tablespoons chopped parsley and the grated rind of 1 lemon and bake in a preheated oven, at 400°F, for 20 minutes, until the vegetables are tender and the fish is opaque and cooked through. Meanwhile, make the tartar sauce as above and serve with the fish and vegetables.

KID-FORA-DOJ

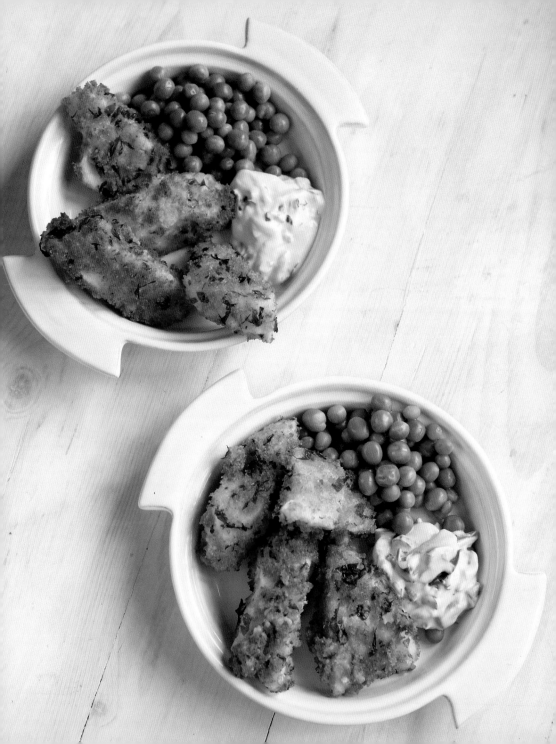

30 Chicken, Bacon, and Leek Pies

Serves 4

1 store-bought rolled dough
  pie crust
beaten egg, to glaze
1 tablespoon olive oil
3 tablespoons butter
12 oz skinless, boneless chicken
  breast, cut into small chunks
8 bacon slices, cut into pieces
2 leeks, rinsed, trimmed, and cut
  into slices
2 tablespoons all-purpose flour
1¼ cups milk
1 teaspoon Dijon mustard
1 cup crème fraîche or light cream
salt and black pepper
green vegetables, to serve

- Line a baking sheet with parchment paper. Cut the pastry into 4 equal rectangles or squares and place on the baking sheet so the pastry is not lying completely flat, lightly brush with beaten egg, and bake in a preheated oven, at 400°F, for 12–15 minutes, until golden.

- Meanwhile, heat the oil and 1 tablespoon of the butter in a heavy skillet and cook the chicken and bacon over high heat for 8–10 minutes, until golden. Add the leeks and cook for 5 minutes. Remove from the heat and set aside.

- Heat the remaining butter in a saucepan and add the flour. Cook for a few seconds, remove from the heat, and add the milk, a little at a time, stirring well after each addition. Add the mustard, return to the heat, and bring to a boil, stirring, until thickened. Add the crème fraîche or light cream and cook for 1–2 minutes. Season, then pour into the skillet with the chicken and stir. Ladle the chicken onto 4 plates, top each with a pastry rectangle, and serve with green veg.

 Chicken, Bacon, and Leek Sauté Cut 2 (6 oz) chicken breasts in half lengthwise. Heat 2 tablespoons butter in a saucepan and cook the pieces over medium heat for 5–6 minutes, turning once, until cooked. Heat 2 tablespoons butter in a skillet and cook 3 coarsely chopped bacon slices and 2 coarsely chopped leeks over high heat for 5 minutes, until soft. Add 1 cup crème fraîche or light cream and 1 teaspoon Dijon mustard and bring to a boil. Spoon the hot sauce over the chicken and serve.

 Chicken, Bacon, and Leeks with Potato Cakes Heat 1 tablespoon olive oil and 1 tablespoon butter in a large, heavy skillet. Cook 12 oz skinless, boneless chicken breast, cut into small chunks, and 8 bacon slices, cut into pieces, for 8–10 minutes, until golden. Add 2 leeks, rinsed, trimmed, and cut into slices, and cook for another 5 minutes, until the leeks are tender and soft. Add 1½ cups canned condensed chicken soup and heat for 5 minutes, until piping hot. Meanwhile, cook 4 prepared potato cakes or hash browns under a preheated hot broiler for 2–3 minutes, until lightly toasted on the top and piping hot. Ladle the chicken and bacon mixture onto warm serving plates and top each with a hot potato cake.

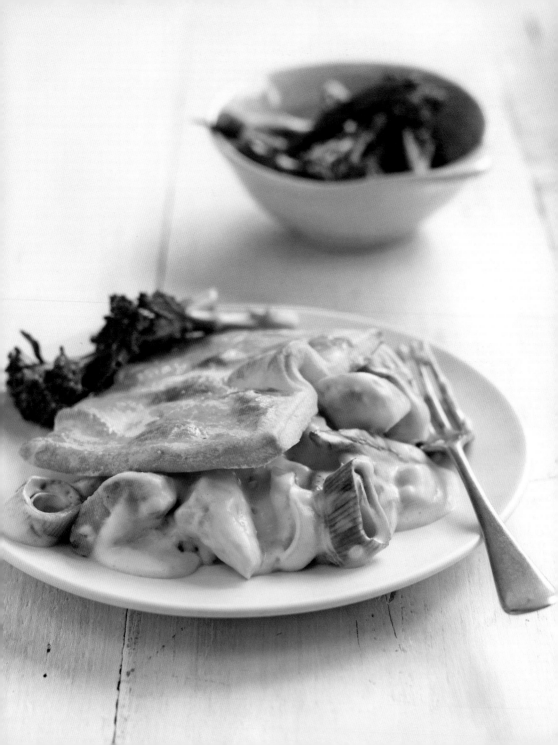

30 Chicken, Chorizo, and Shrimp Jambalaya

Serves 4

1 tablespoon olive oil

6 oz skinless, boneless chicken breast, thinly sliced

4 oz chorizo, thinly sliced

1 red bell pepper, cored, seeded, and coarsely chopped

1 teaspoon Cajun spice

1 cup paella rice or risotto rice

1 (14½ oz) can diced tomatoes

½ cup coarsely chopped okra

4 cups chicken stock

2 oz raw peeled shrimp

warm crusty bread, to serve

- Heat the oil in a large, heavy skillet and cook the chicken, chorizo, and red bell pepper over high heat for 5 minutes, until browned.

- Add the Cajun spice and stir to coat, then add the rice, tomatoes, and okra and stir again. Pour in the stock and bring to a boil, then reduce the heat, cover, and simmer for 20–25 minutes, stirring occasionally, until the rice is tender, adding more water, if necessary.

- Add the shrimp for the final 10 minutes of cooking and stir into the rice to heat through.

- Serve with warm crusty bread.

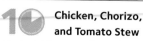 **Chicken, Chorizo, and Tomato Stew**

Heat 1 tablespoon olive oil in a nonstick saucepan and cook 8 oz skinless, boneless chicken breast, cut into small cubes, and 4 oz thinly sliced chorizo over high heat for 5 minutes. Add 1 teaspoon Cajun spice, 2 (14½ oz) cans diced tomatoes, and 1 cup frozen peas. Bring to a boil, then simmer for 3 minutes, until piping hot. Serve ladled over instant rice or instant mashed potatoes.

 Chicken, Shrimp and Chorizo Pilaf

Cook 1 cup instant long grain rice in a large saucepan of lightly salted boiling water according to the package directions, until tender, then drain. Meanwhile, heat 2 tablespoons olive oil in a large, heavy skillet and cook 8 oz thinly sliced chicken breast, 4 oz thinly sliced chorizo, and 1 cored, seeded, and coarsely chopped bell red pepper over high heat for 10 minutes, until cooked and softened. Add 1 teaspoon Cajun spice and stir, then add 1 cup frozen peas and cook for 2 minutes. Add the drained rice and stir-fry for 3–4 minutes, until all the ingredients are piping hot and cooked through.

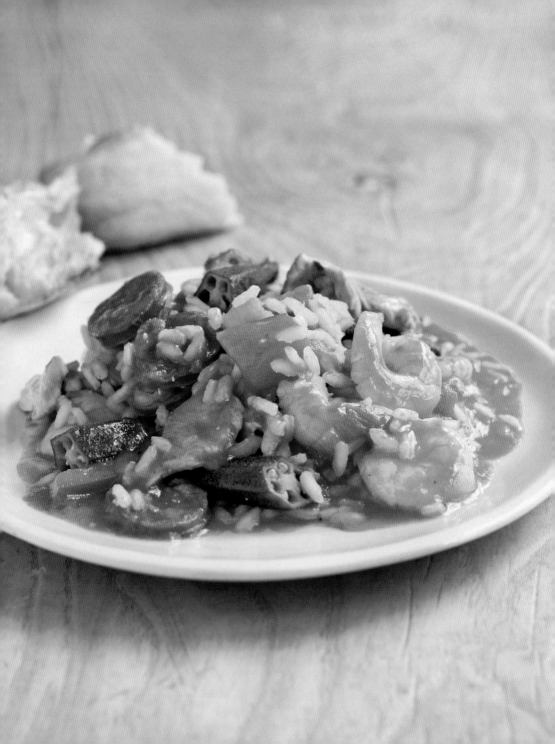

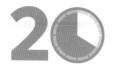 # Pork Dumplings with Dipping Sauce

Serves 4

8 oz ground pork

2 scallions, coarsely chopped

4 canned water chestnuts, coarsely chopped

½ teaspoon ginger paste from a jar or tube

1 tablespoon soy sauce

1 tablespoon teriyaki sauce

24 wonton wrappers

1 tablespoon sunflower oil

½ cup water

For the dipping sauce

3 tablespoons soy sauce

2 tablespoons sweet chili sauce

1 teaspoon sesame oil

juice of ½ lime

- Place the pork, scallions, water chestnuts, ginger paste, soy sauce, and teriyaki sauce in a food processor and pulse to make a coarse paste. Place spoonfuls of the mixture in the center of each wonton wrapper and lightly brush the edges with water. Gather up the edges to make a bundle and pleat the edges a few times to enclose the filling.

- Heat a large, nonstick skillet until hot. Add the oil and arrange the dumplings in a single layer in the skillet (you may have to do this in 2 batches). Cook for 2 minutes, until golden on the bottom, then pour in the measured water. Cover and cook for 6–7 minutes, until the water has been absorbed.

- Mix together the dipping sauce ingredients and serve with the dumplings.

Sticky Pork Mini Wraps

Heat a nonstick skillet or wok until very hot. Add 12 oz ground pork and stir-fry for 5 minutes, until browned and clumpy. Add 2 tablespoons teriyaki sauce and 1 tablespoon sweet chili sauce and continue to cook until the mixture turns sticky. Serve in warmed, thin pancakes (the kind you would use for crispy duck) with sticks of cucumber and extra teriyaki sauce for dipping.

Steamed Pork Dumplings with Chinese Vegetables

Blend 8 oz ground pork with 2 chopped scallions, 4 chopped canned water chestnuts, ½ teaspoon ginger paste, 1 tablespoon soy sauce, and 1 tablespoon teriyaki sauce. Place spoonfuls on 24 wonton wrappers and brush the edges with water. Gather the edges in the middle and scrunch to make purses. Lightly grease 2 bamboo steamer pans and arrange the dumplings in a single layer. Cover and steam for 5–6 minutes. Meanwhile, heat 1 tablespoon sunflower oil in a large wok or skillet, add 3 cups broccoli florets, 2 cups snow peas, and 1 head of bok choy, separated into leaves, and stir-fry for 3 minutes. Add 2 tablespoons sweet chili sauce, 1 tablespoon soy sauce, and 1 tablespoon teriyaki sauce. Bring to a boil, heat through, and serve with the steamed dumplings.

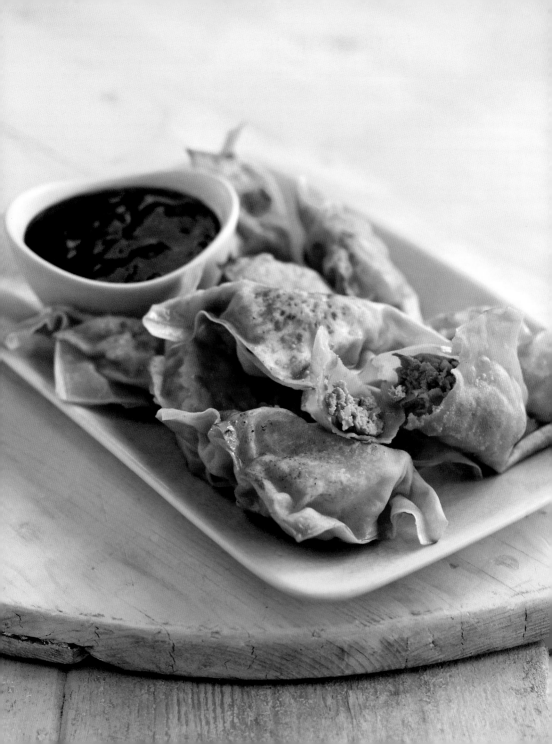

30 Creamy Pesto Fish Pie

Serves 4

1 lb skinless white fish fillets,
  cut into chunks

3 tablespoons pesto

1 cup crème fraîche or light cream

1 sheet ready-to-bake
  puff pastry

beaten egg, to glaze

salt and black pepper

To serve

new potatoes

green beans

- Sprinkle the chunks of fish evenly over the bottom of a shallow ovenproof dish. Stir the pesto into the crème fraîche or light cream in a bowl, then spoon the mixture over the fish. Season with salt and black pepper.

- Unroll the pastry, place it over the dish to cover, and trim off any excess with a sharp knife. Brush the pastry with beaten egg.

- Bake in a preheated oven, at 400°F, for 20–25 minutes, until the pastry is risen and golden and the fish is cooked. Serve with new potatoes and green beans.

10 Creamy Pesto Mackerel Tagliatelle

Cook 1 lb tagliatelle in a saucepan of lightly salted boiling water according to the package directions, until just cooked, then drain and return to the pan. Add 1 cup crème fraîche or light cream, 1 tablespoon pesto, 5 oz flaked cooked mackerel fillets, the juice of ½ lemon, and 2 handfuls of baby spinach leaves. Heat, stirring gently, until the sauce comes to a boil. Season with salt and black pepper and serve.

20 Broiled Creamy Pesto Fish with

Hash Browns Cook 8 small or 4 large frozen prepared hash browns according to the package directions. Meanwhile, place 4 halved tomatoes on a baking sheet and sprinkle with a little grated Parmesan cheese. Bake in the oven. Place 4 (5 oz) pieces of skinless white fish fillet, on an aluminum foil-lined broiler pan that has been lightly oiled. Mix together 4 teaspoons pesto and 3 tablespoons crème fraîche or light cream in a bowl, then spoon the mixture over each piece of fish. Drizzle with a little olive oil and cook under a preheated medium broiler for 8–10 minutes, until the fish is cooked and opaque. Serve with the hash browns and baked tomatoes.

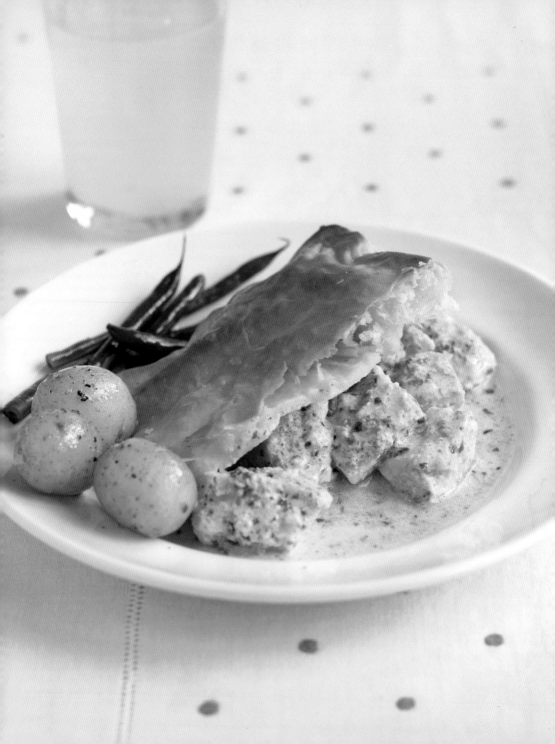

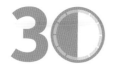

Sticky Chicken Drumsticks with Cucumber and Corn Salad

Serves 4

8 small chicken drumsticks
¼ cup maple syrup
2 tablespoons soy sauce
2 tablespoons sesame oil
½ teaspoon Chinese five spice powder
¼ cucumber, thinly sliced
1 cup drained, canned corn kernels
1 red bell pepper, cored, seeded, and thinly sliced
3 tablespoons prepared French dressing
black pepper

- Make 3 deep slashes in the flesh of each of the chicken pieces. Mix together the maple syrup, soy sauce, sesame oil, and Chinese five spice powder in a large mixing bowl, add the chicken drumsticks, and toss to coat. Transfer to a roasting pan and pour over any of the remaining marinade. Roast in a preheated oven, at 400°F, for 25 minutes, until the chicken is browned and cooked through.

- Meanwhile, make the salad. Place the cucumber, corn kernels, and red bell pepper in a bowl and toss well.

- Add the French dressing and toss well again, seasoning with black pepper. Serve with the hot chicken.

1 Chicken Drumsticks with Sticky Dipping Sauce and Crudités Place 4 cooked chicken drumsticks on a microwave-proof plate. Mix 3 tablespoons maple syrup with 2 tablespoons soy sauce and ½ teaspoon Chinese five spice powder. Brush the mix liberally over the chicken, then heat in a microwave oven for 8 minutes, until piping hot. Meanwhile, cut 1 cored and seeded red bell pepper and ½ cucumber into sticks and place on a serving platter. Mix ¼ cup hoisin sauce with 1 tablespoon maple syrup and place in a bowl in the center of the platter. Serve with the hot drumsticks for dipping.

2 Sticky Chicken and Vegetable Pan-Fry Heat 3 tablespoons sesame oil in a skillet and cook 12 oz thinly sliced chicken breast over high heat for 3 minutes, then add 1 thinly sliced zucchini and 1 cored, seeded, and sliced red bell pepper and cook for another 5–6 minutes, until browned and tender. Meanwhile, mix 3 tablespoons soy sauce with 3 tablespoons honey and ½ teaspoon Chinese five spice powder. Pour into the chicken and continue to cook over a high heat for 1 minute. Add 1 cup drained, canned corn kernels, toss, and cook for another 5 minutes, until piping hot. Serve with instant rice, if desired.

KID-FORA-BOM

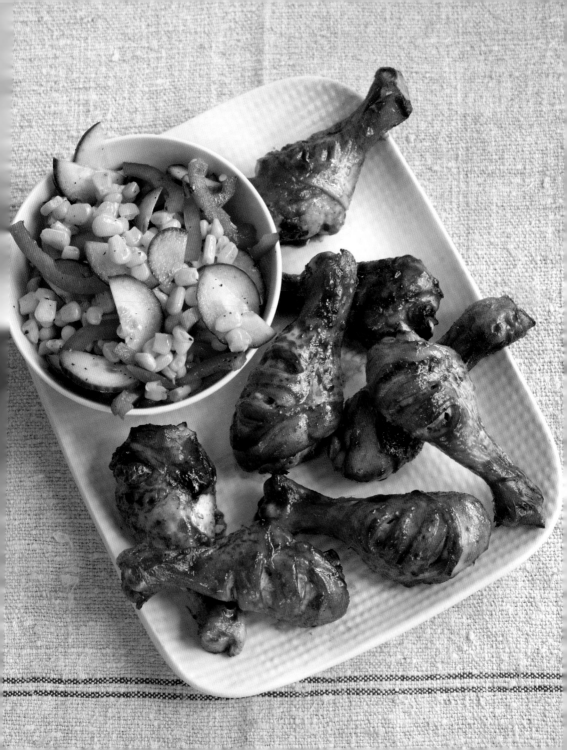

10 Curried Lamb Sandwiches

Serves 4

2 (4 oz) lamb cutlets
  or turkey cutlets
1 teaspoon mild curry powder
2 tablespoons olive oil
4 thick slices of freshly cut
  whole-wheat bread
2 tablespoons mango chutney
handful of salad greens
black pepper

- Place the lamb cutlets or turkey cutlets between 2 sheets of plastic wrap on a board and bash with a rolling pin until half thickness. Remove the plastic wrap and season each side with a little black pepper, then sprinkle each side with the curry powder to lightly coat.

- Heat the oil in a large skillet and cook the lamb over high heat for 3–4 minutes on each side, until cooked through.

- Place the bread slices on a board and top each of 2 slices with 1 tablespoon mango chutney, then top with the hot lamb. Sprinkle with the salad greens, and top each with another slice of bread.

- Cut each sandwich in half diagonally and serve 1 half per child.

 2 Curried Lamb Burgers Place 12 oz ground lamb in a mixing bowl and season with black pepper. Add 1 tablespoon mild curry powder and 3 tablespoons chopped cilantro and mix well, using a fork to mash the flavors together. Using your hands, divide the mixture into 4, then shape each piece into a patty. Place on an aluminum foil-lined broiler rack and lightly brush with oil. Cook under a preheated broiler for 3–4 minutes on each side, until cooked through. Divide among 4 split whole-wheat rolls and top with 1 tablespoon mango chutney and some lettuc. Serve hot with halved cherry tomatoes.

 3 Curried Lamb with Naan Heat a large skillet and cook 1 lb ground lamb or ground turkey and 1 coarsely chopped onion over high heat for 10 minutes, until browned. Add 2 tablespoons mild curry powder and cook for another minute, then add 1¼ cup lamb stock (or chicken stock if using turkey) and 1 (14½ oz) can diced tomatoes. Bring to a boil, then reduce the heat, cover, and simmer for 15 minutes, until the meat is cooked. Stir through 3 tablespoons chopped cilantro. Warm 2 naans in a microwave or hot oven and serve the lamb ladled onto halves of warm naan.

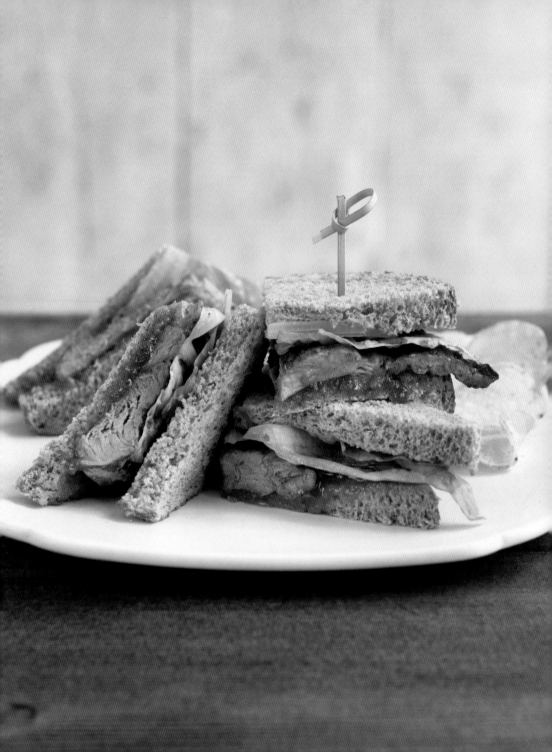

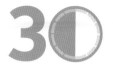

Sticky Pork Ribs with Homemade Baked Beans

Serves 4

2½ lb pork spareribs
¼ cup honey
2 tablespoons soy sauce
2 garlic cloves, crushed
2 tablespoons ketchup
crusty bread, to serve

For the beans

1 tablespoon sunflower oil
1 carrot, peeled and chopped
1 celery stick, chopped
1 (15 oz) can navy beans, rinsed and drained
1 (14½ oz) can diced tomatoes
1 teaspoon paprika
1 teaspoon Worcestershire sauce
pinch of sugar

- Place the spareribs in a large saucepan and cover with boiling water. Cover and simmer for 10 minutes.

- In a small saucepan, gently melt the honey with the soy sauce, garlic, and ketchup. Drain the ribs, place on an aluminum foil-lined baking sheet, and pour the honey mixture over them. Turn to coat evenly, then cook in a preheated oven, at 425°F, for 15 minutes, turning occasionally, until sticky and beginning to char at the edges.

- Meanwhile, make the beans. Heat the oil in a saucepan, add the carrot and celery, and cook, stirring, for 5 minutes to soften. Add the beans, tomatoes, paprika, Worcestershire sauce, and sugar, stir well, and bring to a simmer. Cover and simmer gently for 15 minutes, stirring occasionally.

- Serve the ribs with the beans and crusty bread.

 Sausage and Smoky Bean Baguettes

Broil or fry 4 pork link sausages until cooked through. Heat 1 (15 oz) can baked beans with ½ teaspoon smoked paprika and a dash of Worcestershire sauce in a saucepan. Cut 1 baguette into 4 pieces and split each piece almost in half lengthwise. Butter the bread and fill each piece with a sausage and the baked beans.

 Maple Glazed Pork with Kidney Beans

Brush 8 (3 oz) pork cutlets with maple syrup. Cook under a preheated medium broiler for 8–10 minutes, turning occasionally, until golden, cooked through and starting to char at the edges. Meanwhile, heat 1 tablespoon sunflower oil in a skillet and sauté 1 chopped onion and 1 seeded and chopped green bell pepper for 5 minutes to soften. Add 1 (14½ oz) can diced tomatoes and 1 teaspoon mild chili powder. Bring to a boil, add 1 (15 oz) can red kidney beans, drained and rinsed, cover, and simmer for 10 minutes. Season with salt and black pepper and serve with the maple pork slices and a spoonful of sour cream.

KID-FORA-PUA

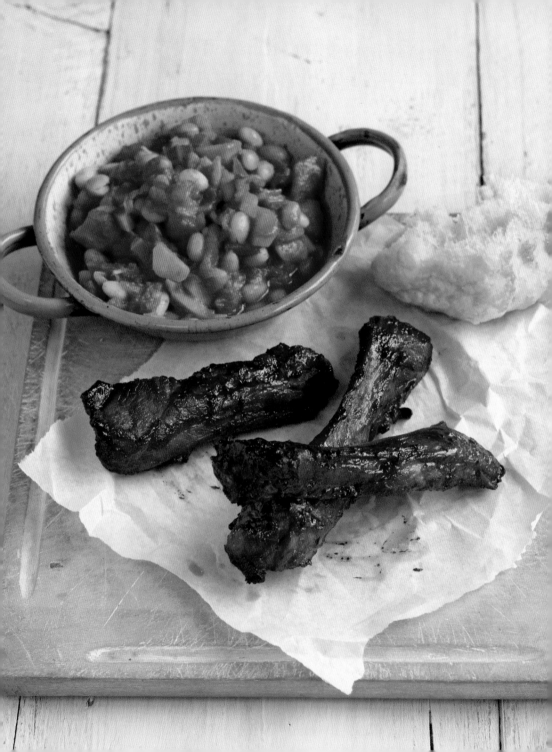

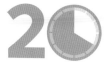

Crispy Chicken with Egg Fried Rice

Serves 4

sunflower oil, for deep frying
⅔ cup all-purpose flour
1 tablespoon cornstarch
1 cup sparkling mineral water
3 boneless, skinless chicken breasts, cut into small chunks

For the fried rice

2 tablespoons sunflower oil
2 bacon slices, chopped
4 scallions, halved and cut into thin strips
1 cup sliced mushrooms
1 (8¾ oz) can corn kernels, drained
½ cup frozen peas
1 cup cooked rice
1 teaspoon Chinese five spice
1 tablespoon soy sauce
2 eggs, beaten

- Fill a wok or deep saucepan halfway with sunflower oil and heat to 350–375°F, or until a cube of bread browns in 30 seconds. Meanwhile, mix together the flour, cornstarch, and a pinch of salt in a bowl. Pour in the sparkling water and mix, using a handheld mixer. Don't overmix—there should still be a few lumps.

- Quickly dip the chicken pieces into the batter, drain off the excess, then add to the hot oil, about 6 pieces at a time. Fry for about 2 minutes, until crisp and browned and the chicken is cooked. Remove with a slotted spoon, drain on paper towels, and keep warm while cooking the remaining chicken.

- To make the fried rice, heat the oil in a large skillet, add the bacon, and cook for 3 minutes, until crisp. Add the scallions, mushrooms, corn, and peas and stir-fry for 2 minutes. Add the rice, Chinese five spice powder, and soy sauce and heat through for 3 minutes, until the rice is hot. Pour in the beaten eggs and stir until cooked.

- Serve the rice with the crispy chicken.

Sweet and Sour Chicken and Rice

Stir-Fry Heat 1 tablespoon sunflower oil in a wok and stir-fry 8 oz thinly sliced chicken breast with 2 chopped bacon slices for 3 minutes. Add ½ (1 lb) package frozen mixed vegetables and 2 cups cooked rice. Stir in ½ cup sweet and sour stir-fry sauce and 1 tablespoon soy sauce and heat through.

Crispy Sweet and Sour Chicken

Mix ⅔ cup all-purpose flour, 1 tablespoon cornstarch, and 1 cup sparking mineral water to make a lumpy batter. Cut 3 boneless, skinless chicken breasts into chunks, dip into the batter, drain off excess, then deep-fry, in batches, in a saucepan filled halfway with sunflower oil heated to 350°F. Fry for 2 minutes, until golden, crisp, and cooked. Drain on paper towels. Heat 1 tablespoon sunflower oil in a wok or skillet and stir-fry 1 chopped onion, 1 carrot, thinly sliced, 1 red bell pepper, seeded and thinly sliced, and 6 baby corn for 2 minutes. Add 1 (8 oz) can pineapple chunks (drained, juice reserved). Heat through. Mix a little of the pineapple juice with 2 tablespoons cornstarch to make a smooth paste. Add the remaining juice, 2 tablespoons tomato sauce, 2 tablespoons vinegar, and 1 tablespoon packed brown sugar to the wok and bring to a boil, stirring, to thicken. Stir in the chicken and serve with rice.

KID-FORA-DUU

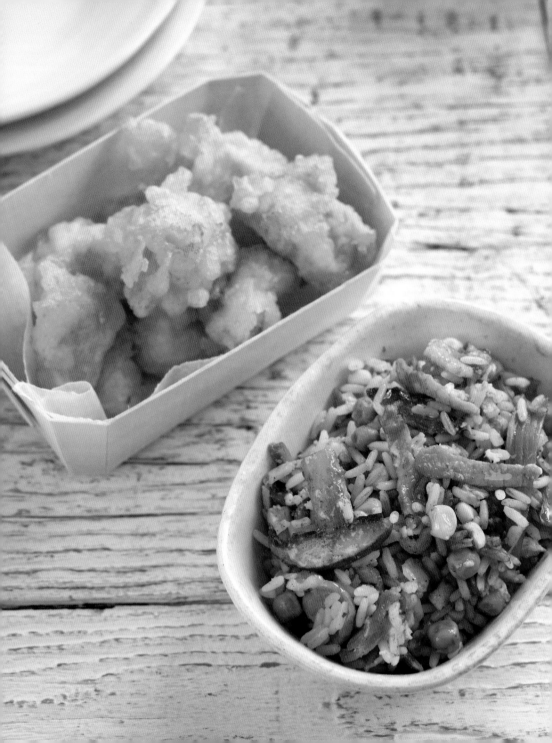

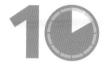

Sausage, Tomato, and Bell Pepper Pan-Fry

Serves 4

1 tablespoon olive oil
24 Vienna sausages or other small sausages, wrapped in bacon
1 each red and yellow bell pepper, cored, seeded, and thinly sliced
½ teaspoon smoked paprika
1 (14½ oz) can diced tomatoes with herbs
cooked long-grain rice or mashed potatoes, to serve

· Heat the oil in a large, heavy skillet and cook the sausages over medium-high heat for 2–3 minutes, until beginning to brown. Add the bell peppers and cook for another 3 minutes, stirring occasionally, until softened.

· Add the smoked paprika and stir well, then add the tomatoes and cook for another 2 minutes, until piping hot and the sausages are cooked through.

· Serve hot over cooked long-grain rice or mashed potatoes.

Smoky Sausage, Tomato, and Bell Pepper Casserole

Cook 12 small sausages under a preheated hot broiler for 10–12 minutes, turning. Heat 2 tablespoons olive oil in a heavy skillet and cook 1 chopped onion for 2 minutes. Add 1 orange and 1 red cored, seeded, and sliced bell pepper and cook for about 3 minutes. Add 1 tablespoon smoked paprika and 6 coarsely chopped tomatoes. Cook for 2 minutes. Add 1¼ cups chicken stock and 1 (15 oz) can cannellini beans, rinsed and drained. Bring to a boil and reduce the heat. Simmer for 3 minutes, add the sausages with the parsley, and stir. Blend 1 tablespoon cornstarch with 3 tablespoons water and add to the skillet, stirring until thickened. Serve with crusty bread.

Sausages and Bell Peppers with Smoky Tomato Gravy Place 8 large sausages in a roasting pan with 2 tablespoons olive oil and toss well to coat. Place in a preheated oven, at 400°F, for 5 minutes. Meanwhile, cut ¼ butternut squash into small pieces and core, seed, and cut 1 red, 1 yellow, and 1 green bell pepper into chunks. Add to the roasting pan with the sausages and toss in the oil, using 2 wooden spoons. Season with black pepper. Return to the oven for 20 minutes, until the vegetables are tender and the sausages are cooked through. Meanwhile, to make the tomato gravy, place ¾ cup canned diced tomatoes in a saucepan with 1¼ cups chicken stock and bring to a boil. Season well with black pepper and add 1 teaspoon Dijon mustard. Transfer to a food processor and process until smooth, then return to the pan and place on the heat. Blend 1 tablespoon cornstarch and ½ teaspoon smoked paprika with 3 tablespoons water and add to the gravy, stirring continuously, until boiled and thickened. Add 1 tablespoon chopped parsley and stir. Serve the sausages and roasted vegetables on warmed serving plates with the tomato gravy spooned over the top.

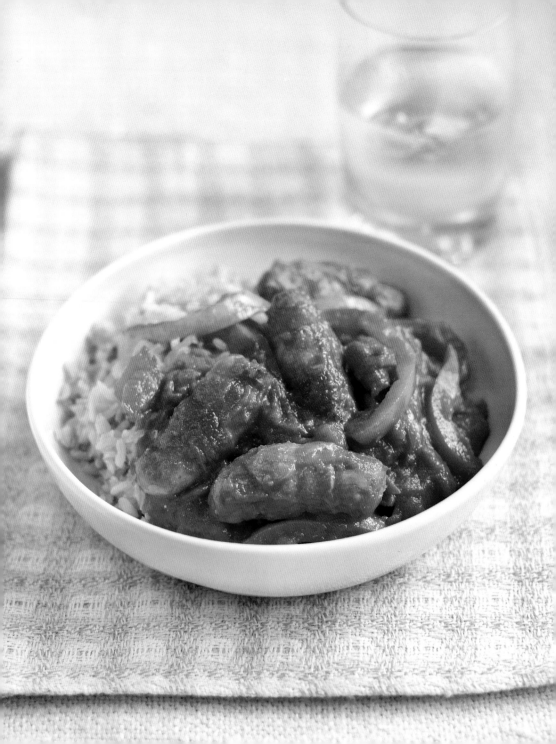

QuickCook
Tasty Treats

Recipes listed by cooking time

3⊙

2⊙

10

10 Strawberry and Raspberry Meringue Desserts

Serves 4

½ cup hulled strawberries, hulled

¾ cup raspberries

2 cups heavy cream

4 small meringue nests, broken into pieces

- Place the strawberries and raspberries in a bowl and lightly crush with a fork.

- Whip the cream in a separate bowl until just thick enough to form soft peaks. Lightly fold in the meringue pieces and the crushed fruit.

- Spoon into glasses or dishes to serve.

20 Hot Berry Meringue Desserts

Using a fork, lightly crush ½ cup hulled strawberries and ¾ cup raspberries with 1 tablespoon confectioners' sugar and spoon into an ovenproof dish. In a clean bowl, whisk 2 egg whites until stiff, then whisk in ⅓ cup superfine sugar, 1 tablespoon at a time, whisking well after each addition until thick and glossy. Spoon the meringue mixture over the fruit and swirl with the back of the spoon. Bake in a preheated oven, at 325°F, for 10 minutes, until golden. Dust with confectioners' sugar and serve immediately.

30 Floating Islands with Raspberries

Heat 2 cups milk in a saucepan until just below boiling point. Meanwhile mix together 1 tablespoon cornstarch, 3 egg yolks, and ⅓ cup superfine sugar. (if you don't have superfine sugar, process the same amount of granulated sugar in a food processor for 1 minute.) Slowly pour the hot milk over the egg yolk mixture, stirring continuously. Pour the mixture back into the pan and cook over medium heat, stirring, until thick enough to coat the back of the spoon. In a separate bowl, whisk 3 egg whites until stiff, then gradually whisk in ⅓ cup superfine sugar. Drop spoonfuls of the meringue mixture into a saucepan of boiling water and cook for about 1 minute, until they float. Remove with a slotted spoon and serve on top of the custard with a few raspberries.

KID-TAST-BUY

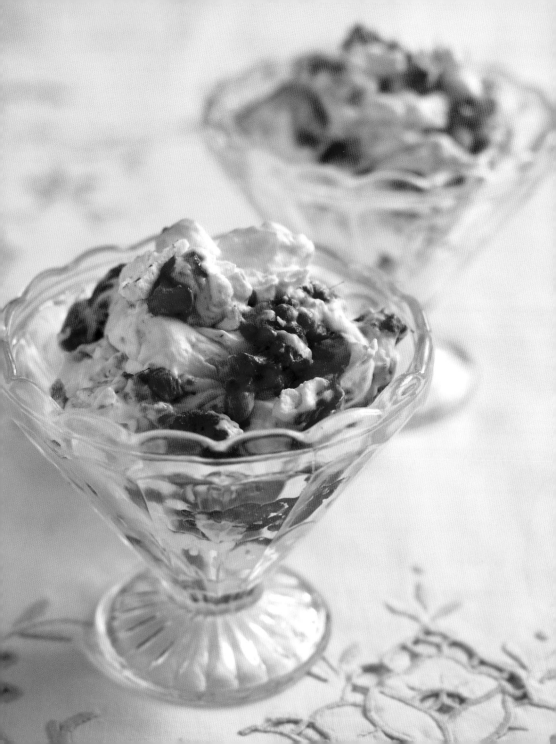

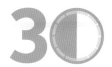 # Peach and Brown Sugar Muffins

Makes 12

2⅓ cups all-purpose flour

2¼ teaspoons baking powder

¾ cup firmly packed light bown sugar, plus extra for sprinkling

½ teaspoon ground allspice

2 ripe peaches, pitted, each cut into 8 wedges and halved horizontally

⅔ cup Greek yogurt

⅔ cup milk

1 extra-large egg

confectioners' sugar, for dusting

- Line a 12-cup muffin pan with paper muffin liners.

- Place the flour, baking powder, sugar, and allspice in a bowl. Chop 20 of the peach pieces and add to the bowl.

- Mix together the yogurt, milk, and egg in small bowl and add to the dry ingredients. Lightly stir until just combined—don't overmix.

- Spoon the batter into the paper liners and push the remaining half wedges of peach into the batter. Sprinkle with a little sugar and bake in a preheated oven, at 375°F, for 15–20 minutes, until well risen and golden. Remove to a wire rack and dust with confectioners' sugar, before serving.

 Peaches and Cream Muffins

Slice 4 prepared muffins each into 3 slices horizontally. Whip ⅔ cup heavy cream with ½ teaspoon ground allspice until just thick enough to form soft peaks, and thinly slice 1 peach. Sandwich the muffins back together with a spoonful of cream and a few slices of peach between the layers.

 Peach and Brown Sugar Croissants

Unroll 1(8 oz) can crescent roll dough and divide into 6 triangles along the perforations. Mix ½ teaspoon ground allspice with ¼ cup demerara sugar or other raw sugar and sprinkle the spiced sugar over the dough. Finely chop 1 ripe peach and sprinkle over the sugar. Roll up the croissants and bake in a preheated oven, at 400°F, for 10–12 minutes, until well risen and golden.

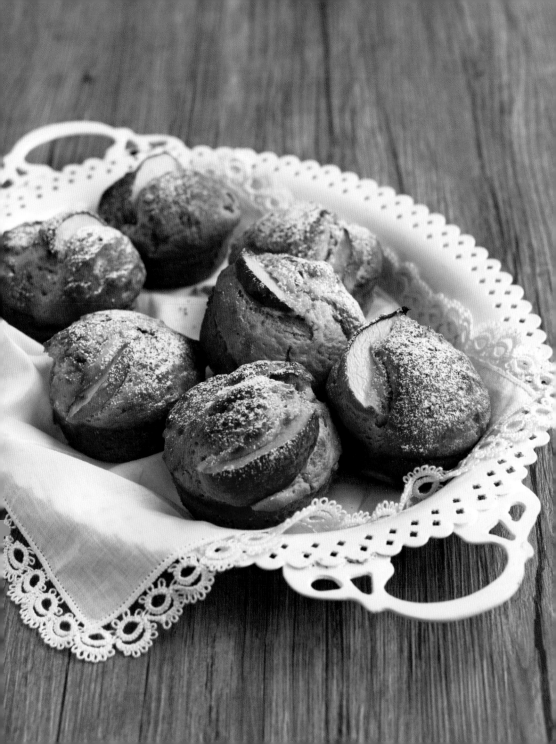

30 Blueberry Scones

Makes 6

2 cups all-purpose flour,
  plus extra for dusting
2 teaspoons baking powder
pinch of salt
4 tablespoons butter
2 tablespoons granulated sugar
1 cup blueberries
2 teaspoons lemon juice
⅔ cup milk, plus extra
  for brushing
honey, to serve

- Line a baking sheet with parchment paper.

- Place the flour, baking powder, and salt in a bowl and rub in the butter using your fingertips until the mixture resembles fine bread crumbs. Stir in the sugar and blueberries.

- Mix the lemon juice with the milk and pour it over the dry ingredients. Quickly mix, using a blunt knife, to form a soft dough, adding a little extra milk if the dough is too dry. Turn out onto a floured surface and lightly knead a few times, then shape into a circle, patting it out with your hands to about ¾ inch thick.

- Cut into 6 wedges, place on the baking sheet, and brush the tops with milk. Bake in a preheated oven, at 425°F, for 10–12 minutes, until well risen and golden.

- Cool slightly and serve warm, halved and spread with honey.

---

1 Blueberry Drop Scones

Beat together 1 cup all-purpose flour, 1 teaspoon baking powder, 2 teaspoons granulated sugar, 1 egg, 1 tablespoon melted butter, and ⅔ cup milk to make a thick batter. Stir in 1 cup blueberries. Drop spoonfuls onto a preheated, lightly greased skillet and cook about 4 at a time for 2 minutes, until bubbles appear. Turn the scones and cook for another minute. Repeat with the remaining mixture. Serve warm with maple syrup.

2 Blueberry Scone Twists

Place 1½ (7½ oz) packages biscuit mix in a bowl. Stir in 1 cup (4 oz) blueberries and make the dough with milk according to the package directions. Knead very lightly, then pat out the dough with your hands on a floured surface to a square about ½ inch thick. Sprinkle the surface with 2 tablespoons demerara sugar or other raw sugar and cut into 8 strips. Twist the strips and place on a baking sheet lined with parchment paper. Lightly brush with milk and bake in a preheated oven, at 425°F, for 10–12 minutes, until well risen and golden. Serve warm or cold.

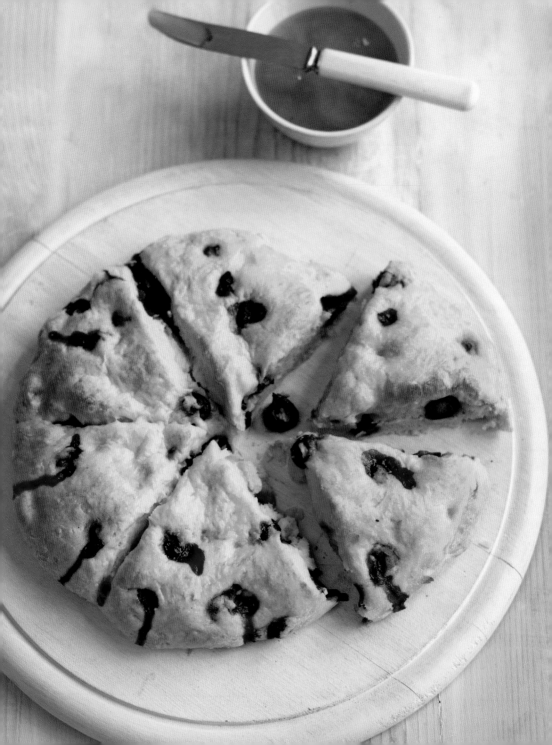

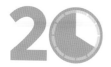

Whole-Wheat Crepes with Peaches and Ice Cream

Serves 4

1 cup whole-wheat flour (or half
  whole-wheat and half
  all-purpose white flour)
pinch of salt
1 egg
1 tablespoon butter, melted
⅔ cup milk
sunflower oil, for frying
3 ripe peaches, pitted and sliced,
  or sliced canned peaches
4 scoops of vanilla ice cream
¼ cup maple syrup

- Place the flour and salt in a mixing bowl. Make a well in the center and break the egg into it. Add the melted butter and one-quarter of the milk. Mix with a wooden spoon or handheld mixer, adding more milk as the batter thickens until all the milk is used. Beat well to make a smooth batter.

- Heat a small, nonstick skillet until hot and lightly grease with a little sunflower oil. Pour in about 2 tablespoons of batter, swirling the skillet so the batter evenly coats the bottom of the skillet. Cook for 1 minute, until golden underneath, then turn over and cook the other side until golden. Slide out onto a plate and keep warm. Repeat with the remaining batter to make 8 thin pancakes.

- Fold the pancakes into quarters and serve with the peach slices, a scoop of ice cream, and a drizzle of maple syrup.

Waffles with Caramel Peaches and Cream

Heat 4 tablespoons butter, ¾ cup firmly packed light brown sugar, and 1 (5 oz) can evaporated milk in a small saucepan until the butter has melted and the sugar dissolved. Bring to a boil and simmer gently for 3 minutes until the mixture has thickened slightly. Stir in 2 sliced peaches and serve with warmed prepared waffles and a spoonful of whipped cream.

Peach Popovers

Beat together 1 cup all-purpose flour, a pinch of salt, 1 egg, 1 cup milk, and 2 tablespoons granulated sugar to make a smooth batter. Place 1 teaspoon sunflower oil in each cup of a 12-cup nonstick muffin pan and heat in a preheated oven, at 425°F, for 5 minutes. Cut 1 peach into 12 wedges and place a wedge of peach in each muffin cup. Quickly pour in the batter, dividing it equally among the cups, and cook in the oven for 15 minutes, until well risen, crisp, and golden. Turn out of the cups and serve warm, drizzled with maple syrup, with a scoop of ice cream.

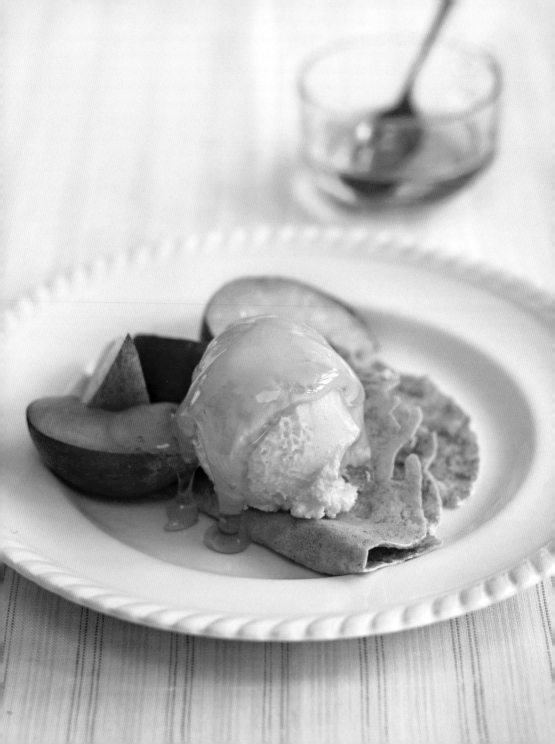

10 Chocolate Desserts with Hidden Prunes

Serves 4

4 oz semisweet chocolate, broken into pieces, plus extra shavings to decorate

2 cups canned prunes in apple juice, drained

1¼ cups Greek yogurt

raspberries, to decorate

- Place the chocolate in a small microwave-proof bowl and melt in a microwave on medium for 1 minute. Stir and return to the microwave, checking every 20 seconds, until melted and smooth.

- Remove the pits from the prunes and process the flesh in a food processor or with a handheld blender until smooth. Stir together the prune puree, yogurt, and chocolate until evenly mixed.

- Spoon into cups or glasses and decorate with chocolate shavings and some raspberries.

 ## Chocolate and Prune Whips

Cook 15 pitted dried prunes in ½ cup apple juice in a small saucepan for 5 minutes, until soft. Puree with a handheld blender until smooth. Stir through 1 cup plain or Greek yogurt with 2 oz melted semisweet chocolate. Layer in glasses, alternating with 1¾ cups prepared vanilla pudding.

 ## Hot Chocolate Prune Puddings

Using an electric mixer, beat together 1 stick softened butter and ⅓ cup firmly packed light brown sugar until soft. Gradually whisk in 2 eggs, 8 oz melted semisweet chocolate, and ½ cup heavy cream. Lightly fold in 2 tablespoons all-purpose flour, ¼ teaspoon baking powder, and 1 cup chopped, pitted dried prunes. Spoon the batter into 4 microwave-proof buttered ramekin dishes. Cover with plastic wrap and microwave on full power for 3–4 minutes, until lightly set. Pierce the plastic wrap and let stand for 2 minutes before turning out. Serve warm with cream.

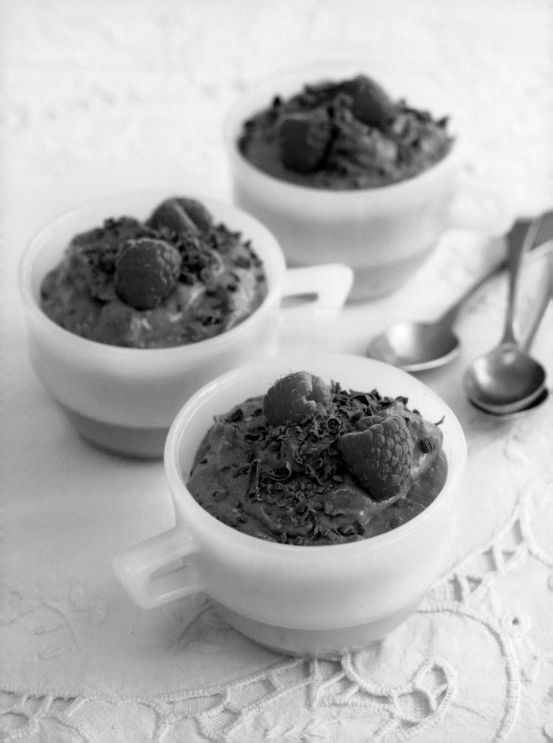

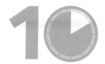 # Fruit and Yogurt Baskets

Serves 4

2 tablespoons honey
1¼ cups Greek yogurt
4 brandy snap baskets
2 cups mixed fruits, such as
strawberries, kiwifruit, apricots,
and grapes, halved or chopped,
depending on the fruit

- Lightly swirl the honey through the yogurt and spoon into the brandy snap baskets.

- Arrange the fruits on top and serve.

 Fruity Yogurt Trifles Using a fork, lightly crush 1 cup hulled strawberries and 1 cup blueberries. Sprinkle with 2 teaspoons confectioners' sugar and let stand for 5 minutes, until juicy. Break 8 ladyfinger cookies into pieces and place in the bottom of 4 glasses or dishes. Spoon the crushed fruit on top with the juice and top with 1 sliced banana. Swirl 2 tablespoons honey into 1¼ cups Greek yogurt and spoon it over the fruit. Decorate with strawberry slices and blueberries.

 Fruit and Yogurt Whips with Homemade Cookies Beat 1 stick softened butter and ¼ cup granulated sugar in a food processor. Add 1⅓ cups all-purpose flour and 1¼ teaspoons baking powder and process until the mixture just comes together and forms a dough. Divide the dough into 12 balls, place on a baking sheet lined with parchment paper, and flatten with the back of a wet fork. Bake in a preheated oven, at 375°F, for 10–12 minutes. Meanwhile, blend 1 cup hulled strawberries and 1 cup blueberries in a food processor until almost smooth. Fold into ⅔ cup Greek yogurt, ½ cup prepared vanilla pudding, and 2 tablespoons honey to create a rippled effect. Spoon into glasses or bowls and serve with the cookies.

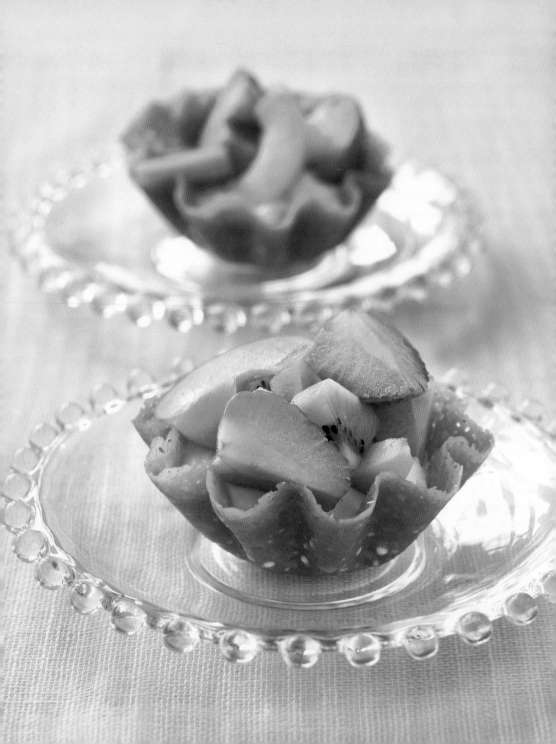

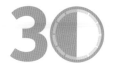

Apricot Oat Bars

Makes 15

2 sticks butter, plus extra
   for greasing
¾ cup light corn syrup
¾ cup firmly packed light
   brown sugar
4 cups rolled oats
½ cup crunchy mixed-grain cereal
1½ cups chopped dried apricots

- Grease a shallow 7 x 11 inch nonstick baking pan.

- Place the butter, corn syrup, and sugar in a large saucepan and heat gently, stirring, until the butter has melted.

- Add the oats, cereal, and apricots and stir well to mix. Transfer the dough into the baking pan and spread evenly.

- Bake in a preheated oven, at 350°F, for 15–20 minutes, until golden. Cut into 15 bars, cool slightly, then remove from the pan. The bars can be stored in an airtight container for up to 5 days.

Apricot and Fig Nibbles

Put 1 cup dried apricots in a food processor with ½ cup dried figs and pulse until chopped. Transfer the chopped fruit to a bowl and stir in 3 cups bran flakes, 1 cup dried flaked coconut, 1 cup condensed milk, and 6 tablespoons butter, melted. Spoon into 16 paper cake liners and eat or chill until set.

Apricot Muesli Cookies

Melt 1 stick butter in a saucepan with 1 tablespoon light corn syrup. Mix 1 teaspoon baking soda with 2 tablespoons boiling water and add to the pan. Pour this mixture onto 2 cups muesli, ¾ cup all-purpose flour, ½ cup granulated sugar, and 1 cup chopped apricots. Stir well, then place 20 small tablespoonfuls of the dough, allowing room for them to spread, on baking sheets lined with parchment paper. Bake in a preheated oven, at 350°F, for 8–10 minutes.

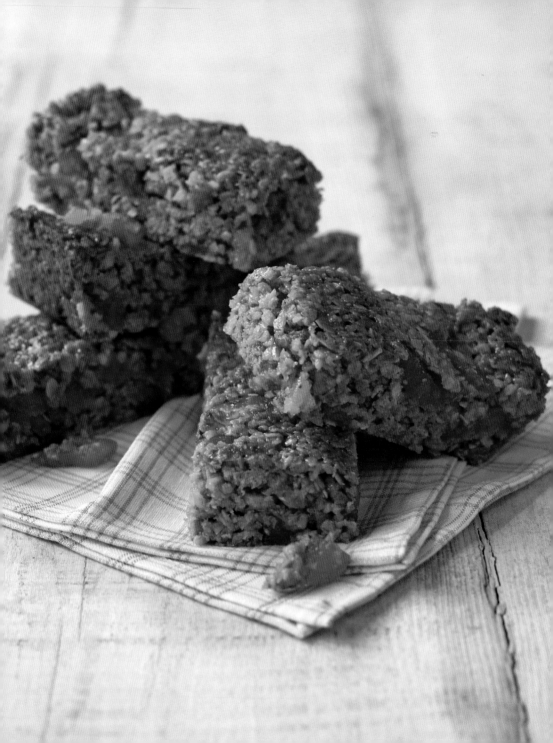

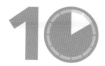

Strawberry Ice Cream Sundae

Serves 4

1 pint strawberries,
  hulled and quartered
⅓ cup confectioners' sugar
8 scoops of vanilla ice cream
1 cup miniature marshmallows
sprinkles, to decorate

- Blend half the strawberries with the confectioners' sugar, using a handheld blender or food processor, until smooth.

- Put 1 scoop of ice cream in the bottom of each of 4 tall glasses, top with half the remaining quartered strawberries, spoon over half the strawberry puree, and sprinkle with half the marshmallows.

- Repeat the layers and finish with some sprinkles. Serve immediately.

2 Strawberry S'mores

Thinly slice 4 hulled strawberries and arrange on the top of 4 chocolate chip cookies. Arrange mini marshmallows in a single layer on the top and cover each with another cookie. Wrap each cookie sandwich in aluminum foil, place on a baking sheet, and bake in a preheated oven, at 350°F, for 5–8 minutes, until the cookies are warm and the marshmallows have started to melt. Serve warm with a scoop of ice cream.

3 Mini Baked Alaskas

Place 4 graham crackers on a baking sheet lined with parchment paper. Top each cookie with a scoop of strawberry ice cream and place in the freezer. Whisk 2 egg whites in a large, clean bowl until stiff enough to form soft peaks. Gradually whisk in ⅔ cup superfine sugar, 1 tablespoon at a time, whisking well after each addition until thick and glossy. Quickly spread and swirl the meringue over the ice cream and cookies, making sure the ice cream is completely covered. Bake in a preheated oven, at 425°F, for 3–4 minutes, until the meringue is golden. Dust with confectioners' sugar and serve immediately before the ice cream starts to melt.

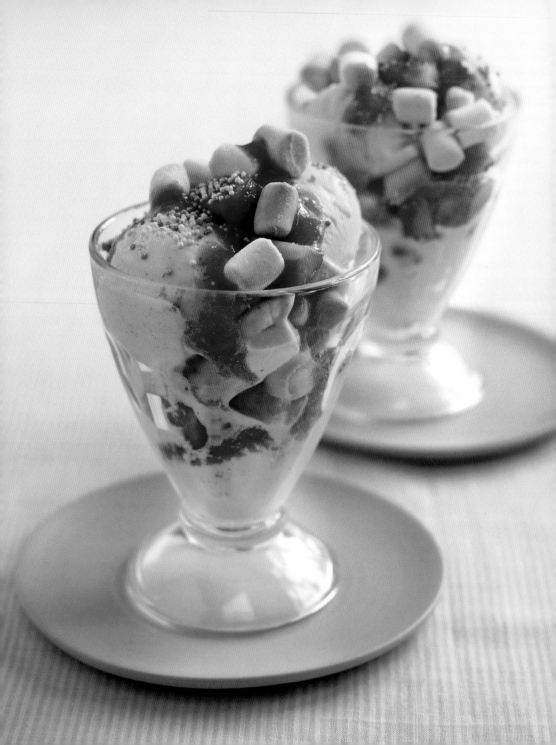

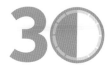

Mango Krispie Cakes

Makes 16

4 tablespoons butter

3 tablespoons light corn syrup

1 tablespoon packed light
brown sugar

3 cups Rice Krispies or
similar cereal

⅔ cup dried mango

⅓ cup raisins

2 tablespoons pumpkin seeds

3 tablespoons sunflower seeds

- Melt the butter in a large saucepan over low heat. Stir in the corn syrup and sugar and stir to dissolve the sugar.

- Remove from the heat, add the Rice Krispies, mango, raisins, pumpkin seeds, and sunflower seeds and stir well to mix.

- Spoon the batter into 16 paper cake liners and chill in the refrigerator for 15 minutes to set.

 Fruit, Seed, and Krispie Mix

Mix together 3 cups Rice Krispies or similar cereal, ⅔ cup chopped dried mango, ⅓ cup raisins, 2 tablespoons pumpkin seeds, and 2 tablespoons sunflower seeds. Sprinkle over ice cream or yogurt, or simply eat as it is.

 Caramel Krispie Cakes

Unwrap 7 oz of caramel candies and place in a saucepan with ¼ cup heavy cream. Slowly melt over low heat, stirring occasionally, until smooth. Stir in 6 cups Rice Krispies or similar cereal and ⅓ cup chopped dried mango until evenly coated. Spoon into 20 paper cake liners.

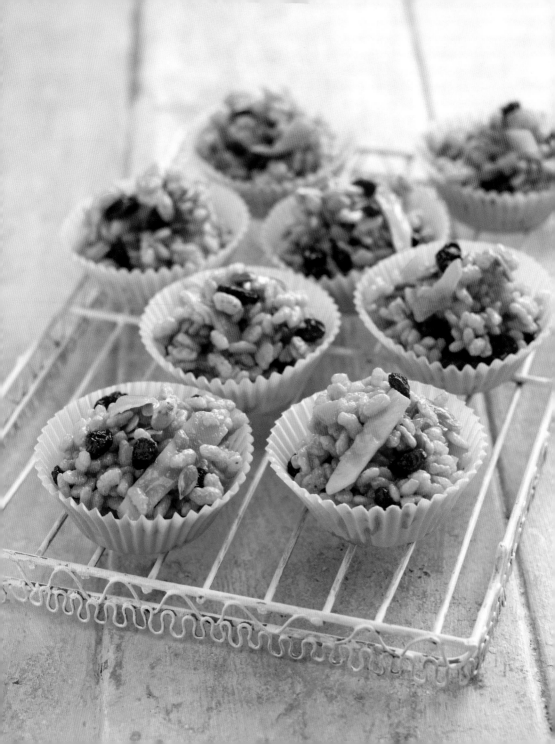

10 Caramel Bananas

Serves 4

2 tablespoons butter

4 bananas, peeled and halved lengthwise

⅓ cup caramel sauce, such as dulce de leche

⅓ cup heavy cream

ice cream, to serve

- Melt the butter in a large skillet. Add the bananas and cook for 2 minutes, turning once, until just starting to soften and brown. Remove from the skillet and place in serving dishes.

- Heat the caramel sauce and cream in the skillet and simmer for 1 minute, until bubbling. Let cool slightly.

- Drizzle the sauce over the bananas and serve with scoops of ice cream.

 Banana Fritters with Caramel Sauce For the caramel sauce, heat 1 stick butter and ⅔ cup firmly packed light brown sugar in a saucepan until the butter has melted and the sugar dissolved. Add ½ cup light cream and simmer for a few minutes, until smooth and golden. Remove from the heat. For the fritters, mix together 1 cup all-purpose flour, 1 teaspoon baking powder, 1 teaspoon baking soda, 2 eggs, and a splash of sparkling mineral water to make a smooth batter. Diagonally slice 2 large bananas and dip into the batter. Shake off the excess and cook, in batches, in a saucepan filled halfway with hot sunflower oil for 2–3 minutes, until crisp and golden. Remove from the pan with a slotted spoon and drain on paper towels. Serve warm with the caramel sauce.

 Banana Caramel Pie Crush 8 oz chocolate-coated graham crackers in a food processor, then mix with 6 tablespoons melted butter. Press the cookie mixture over the bottom and up the sides of a greased 8 inch round tart pan. Arrange 2 sliced bananas over the cookie crust and cover with 1⅔ cups caramel sauce, such as dulce de leche. Whip 1¼ cups heavy whipping cream until just thick enough to form soft peaks, then swirl over the top of the caramel using the back of a spoon. Sprinkle grated chocolate over the top. Chill for 10 minutes to set before serving.

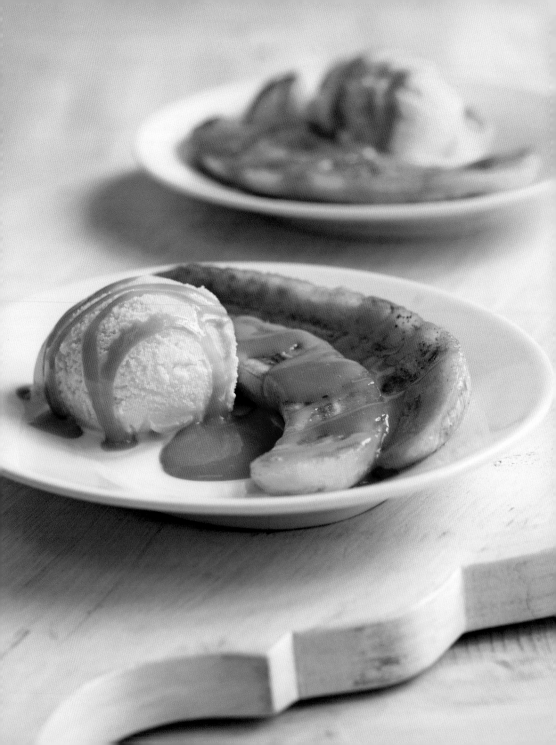

1 Rice Pudding Brûlée

Serves 4

4 tablespoons strawberry or raspberry preserves or jam

2 tablespoons orange juice

1 (22 oz) container prepared rice pudding

⅓ cup demerara sugar or other raw sugar

- Mix together the preserves or jam and orange juice and spoon into the bottom of 4 heatproof dishes.

- Spoon the rice pudding over the top and sprinkle evenly with the sugar.

- Place the puddings under a preheated hot broiler, as near to the heat as possible, and broil for 2–3 minutes, until the sugar is melted and bubbling. Let stand for a few minutes for the topping to cool and set before eating.

 2 Caramelized Blackberry Yogurt Desserts Place 1 cup blackberries in a bowl and mash with a fork until broken into chunky pieces. Add the finely grated rind and juice of 1 orange and 1 tablespoon granulated sugar and stir to mix. Divide among four ¾ cup individual heatproof dishes. Whip ⅔ cup heavy cream until just thick enough to form soft peaks, then stir in 1 cup Greek yogurt. Spoon the yogurt over the blackberries and level the tops just below the rim of each dish. Sprinkle 2 tablespoons granulated sugar evenly over the top of each dish. Place under a preheated hot broiler, as near to the heat as possible, and broil for 2–3 minutes, until the sugar melts and turns golden, making sure it doesn't burn. Let cool until the caramelized topping has set and cooled before serving.

 3 Honey Baked Fruit with Brûlée Topping Cut 4 ripe peaches in half and place in an ovenproof dish with 16 blackberries or 8 hulled strawberries, halved if large. Dot with a little butter and drizzle with 2 tablespoons honey. Bake in a preheated oven, at 375°F, for 20 minutes, until softened. Spoon 1 cup mascarpone cheese over the top, sprinkle with ⅓ cup demerara sugar or other raw sugar, and cook under a preheated hot broiler until the sugar starts to melt and bubble. Cool for 5 minutes before serving.

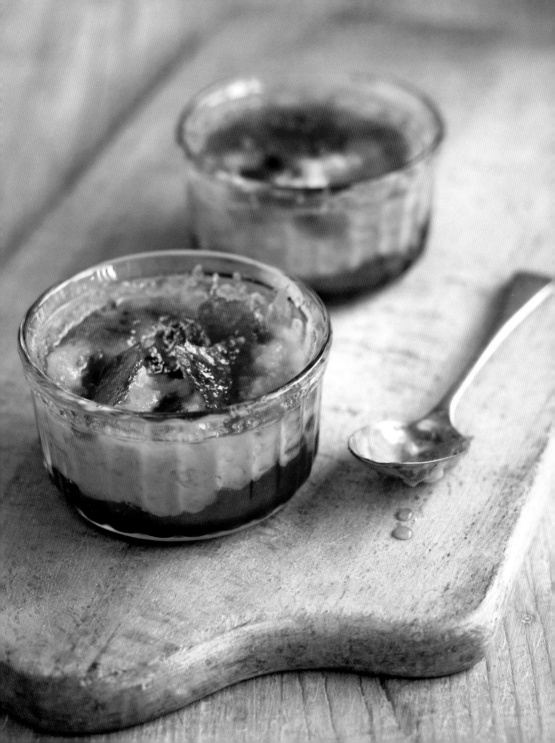

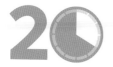

Rhubarb and Strawberry Oat Crisp

Serves 4

1 lb rhubarb, trimmed and cut into ½ inch chunks

3 tablespoons water

6 tablespoons butter

2 cups rolled oats

⅓ cup demerara sugar or other raw sugar

¼ cup strawberry preserves or jam

1 cup hulled and sliced strawberries

prepared vanilla pudding or whipped cream, to serve

- Place the rhubarb in a saucepan with the measured water and cook for 5 minutes, until soft.

- Meanwhile, in a separate saucepan, melt the butter, then stir in the oats and sugar.

- Stir the presevers into the rhubarb, add the sliced strawberries, then transfer to an ovenproof dish. Sprinkle with the oat mixture and bake in a preheated oven, at 400°F, for 15 minutes, until golden.

- Serve warm with vanilla pudding or whipped cream.

---

10 **Rhubarb and Mixed Berry Shortcake Crisps** Cut 10 oz rhubarb into ½ inch chunks and cook in a saucepan with 2 tablespoons butter for 5 minutes, stirring occasionally, until softened. Stir in 1 (16 oz) container prepared mixed berry compote and heat through. Spoon into bowls and sprinkle with 1½ cups crumbled shortcake cookies. Serve warm with cream.

30 **Nutty Rhubarb and Strawberry Crisp** Cut 1 lb rhubarb into ½ inch chunks and place in a large baking dish with 2 cups hulled and halved strawberries. Sprinkle with ⅓ cup granulated sugar and bake in a preheated oven, at 400°F, for 10 minutes. Meanwhile, place 1⅓ cups all-purpose flour in a food processor with 1 stick butter and ⅓ cup demerara sugar or other raw sugar. Pulse until the mixture forms fine bread crumbs. Transfer to a bowl and stir in ⅔ cup chopped hazelnuts. Rub the crumbs together until they start to form clumps, sprinkle them over the fruit, and return to the oven for 15 minutes, until the crisp is golden. Serve warm with cream.

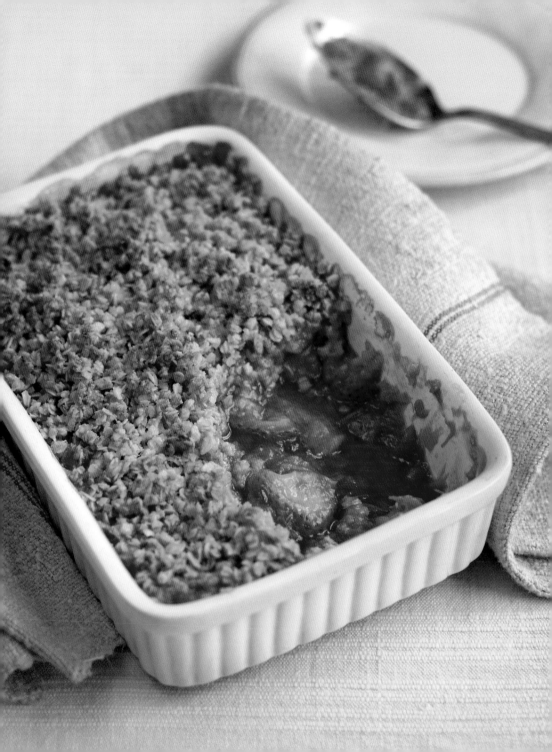

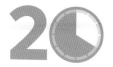

White Chocolate and Apricot Squares

Makes 9

8 oz white chocolate, broken into pieces

2 cups Rice Krispies or similar cereal

⅓ cup chopped dried apricots

- Line a shallow 8 inch square baking pan with plastic wrap.

- Heat 6 oz of the white chocolate in a heatproof bowl over a saucepan of simmering water, making sure the bottom of the bowl doesn't touch the water. Let heat for a few minutes, stirring occasionally, until the chocolate is melted and smooth.

- Remove the bowl from the pan and stir the Rice Krispies and apricots into the melted chocolate. Spoon the mixture into the prepared pan and press down firmly. Chop the remaining 2 oz chocolate and sprinkle over the top. Place in the freezer for 15 minutes to chill and set.

- Cut into 9 squares to serve.

White Chocolate and Apricot Popcorn Stir 1 (4 oz) unsalted buttered popcorn into 3 oz melted white chocolate with ⅓ cup chopped dried apricots. Spoon into small paper cones or cupcake liners and chill in the freezer for 5 minutes to set.

White Chocolate and Fruit Refrigerator Cake Melt 7 oz white chocolate, broken into pieces, 6 tablespoons butter, and 2 tablespoons light corn syrup in a heatproof bowl over a saucepan of simmering water. Stir until melted, then remove from the heat and stir in 10 broken graham crackers, 1 cup cornflakes, ⅓ cup raisins, ⅔ cup chopped dried apricots, and ⅓ cup dried cranberries. Mix well, then spoon into a shallow 8 inch square cake pan lined with plastic wrap. Place in the freezer for 20 minutes to chill and set. Cut into squares.

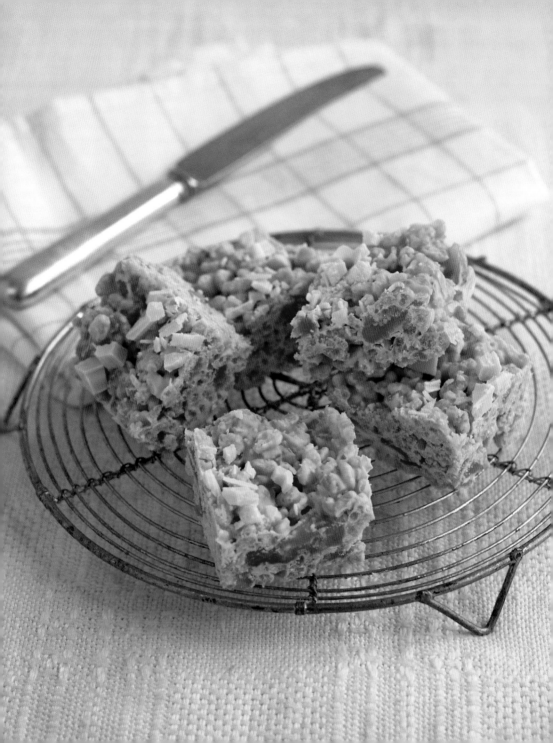

30 Apple and Almond Tart

Serves 6

1 sheet ready-to-bake
  puff pastry
8 oz marzipan, coarsely grated
2 Pippin apples, cored and
  thinly sliced
¼ cup apricot preserves, warmed
½ cup slivered almonds
cream or ice cream, to serve

- Unroll the puff pastry and place on a baking sheet. Sprinkle the grated marzipan evenly over the pastry, then arrange the apple slices in rows over the top.

- Brush the apricot preserves over the apple slices and sprinkle with the slivered almonds. Bake in a preheated oven, at 400°F, for 20 minutes, until the pastry is golden and cooked.

- Cut into squares and serve warm with cream or ice cream.

---

1 **Speedy Apple Pies**
Heat 12 oz prepared apple slices in 2 tablespoons butter in a skillet, add ½ teaspoon ground cinnamon and ¼ cup golden raisins, and heat through, adding a little water, if necessary. Spoon into dishes and place 1 prepared palmier pastry on top of each. Serve with cream.

2 **Hot Apple Slices with Cinnamon Pastries** Unroll 1 sheet ready-to-bake puff pastry. Mix ¼ cup granulated sugar and 1 teaspoon ground cinnamon and sprinkle evenly over the pastry. Starting along one of the long sides, loosely roll the pastry into a long roll. Cut into ½ inch slices and lay flat on 2 baking sheets lined with parchment paper. Sprinkle with a little extra sugar and bake in a preheated oven, at 400°F, for 10 minutes, until golden and crisp. Meanwhile, cook 3 cored and sliced Pippin apples in 2 tablespoons butter for 5 minutes, until softened and starting to brown. Add ¼ cup golden raisins. Serve with the cinnamon pastries.

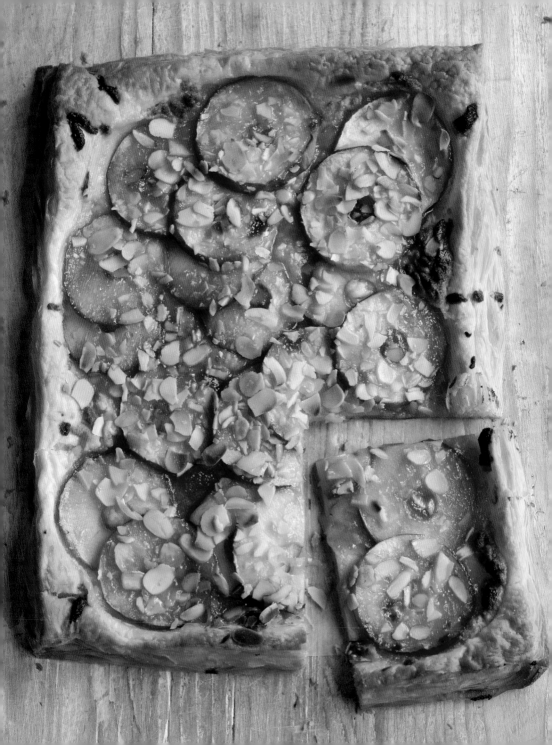

30 Strawberry and Lime Cheesecakes

Serves 4

1 cup crushed oatmeal cookies
4 tablespoons butter, melted
⅓ cup condensed milk
1 cup mascarpone cheese
finely grated rind and juice
 of 1 lime
1 cup hulled and sliced
 strawberries
1 tablespoon strawberry
 preserves or jam

- Mix together the crushed cookies and butter and spoon into the bottom of 4 chunky glasses or ramekins. Press down firmly with the back of a small spoon.

- In a bowl, mix the condensed milk and mascarpone until soft and creamy. Stir in the lime rind and juice and spoon into the glasses.

- Mix together the strawberries and preserves (if the preserves are very thick, soften them with a splash of boiling water) and spoon over the top of the cheesecakes.

---

10 Strawberry and Lime Cheesecake

Stacks Mix 1 cup mascarpone cheese with ½ cup condensed milk and stir in the grated rind and juice of 1 lime. Spoon half the mascarpone mixture onto 4 graham crackers and top with ½ cup sliced, hulled strawberries. Repeat the layers and finish with a dusting of confectioners' sugar.

20 Strawberry and Lime Tiramisu

Place 8 ladyfingers in a single layer in the bottom of a dish. Arrange ½ cup sliced, hulled strawberries over the top and dust generously with confectioners' sugar. Mix together 1 cup mascarpone cheese, ½ cup condensed milk, and the grated rind and juice of 1 lime. Spread half the mixture over the strawberries, cover with 8 more ladyfingers, another ½ cup sliced, hulled strawberries, and a dusting of confectioners' sugar. Spoon the remaining mascarpone mixture over the top, sprinkle with 1 oz grated chocolate, and decorate with extra strawberries.

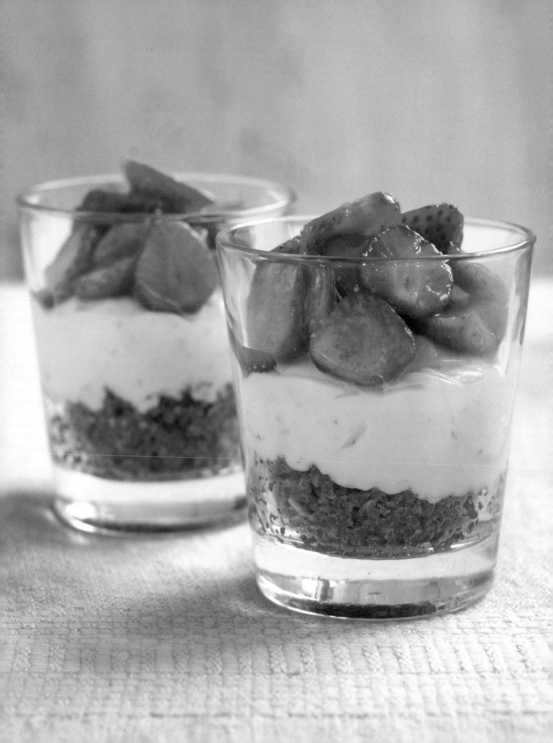

30 Orange Drizzle Sheet Cake

Makes 12

½ cup packed sunflower spread

⅔ cup granulated sugar,
   plus ¼ cup

1 cup all-purpose flour

1 teaspoon baking powder

2 eggs

finely grated rind and juice of
   1 orange

crystallized orange and lemon
   slices, to decorate

- Line a shallow 7 x 11 inch baking pan with parchment paper.

- Place the sunflower spread, ⅔ cup sugar, flour, baking powder, eggs, and orange rind in a mixing bowl and beat with an electric mixer until soft and creamy. Spoon the batter into the pan and spread the surface level.

- Bake in a preheated oven, at 350°F, for 20 minutes, until risen and just firm to the touch. Meanwhile, mix together the orange juice and remaining sugar in a bowl. Remove the cake from the oven and drizzle the mixture over the cake.

- Cut into 12 fingers or squares and top each with a crystallized orange and lemon slice.

---

1 Sticky Orange Syrup Cakes

Heat ¼ cup marmalade in a small saucepan with 2 tablespoons water until melted, then bring to a boil. Remove from the heat and strain with a strainer. Spoon the syrup over 12 prepared plain cupcakes and let soak for a few minutes. Dust with confectioners' sugar to serve.

2 Iced Orange Cupcakes

Using an electric mixer, beat ½ cup packed sunflower spread, ⅔ cup granulated sugar, 1 cup all-purpose flour, 1 teaspoon baking powder, 2 eggs, and 2 tablespoons orange marmalade until soft and creamy. Spoon into 12 paper cake liners and bake in a preheated oven, at 350°F, for 10 minutes, until risen and just firm to the touch. Meanwhile, mix together 1¼ cups confectioners' sugar, the finely grated rind of ½ orange, and enough orange juice to make a smooth, thick icing. Spoon the icing over the cakes.

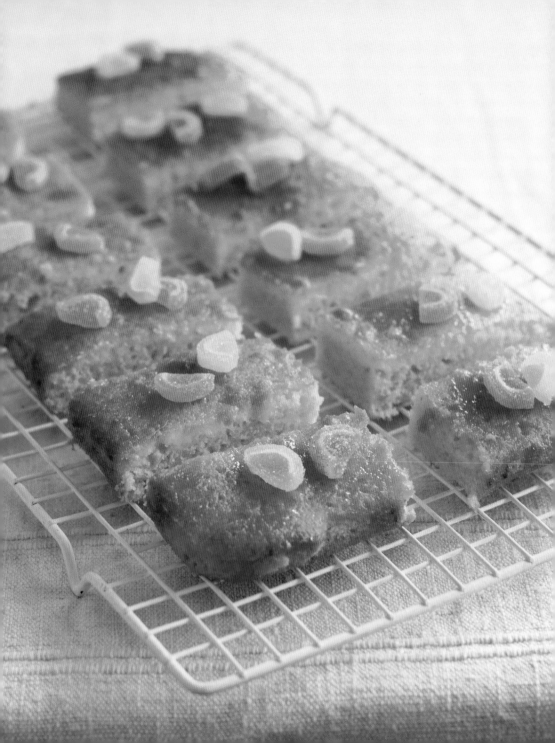

30 Cherry Clafouti

Serves 4

1 (15 oz) can pitted black
cherries, drained and dried
on paper towels

1 cup all-purpose flour

¼ cup granulated sugar

3 eggs

1¾ cups milk

confectioners' sugar, for dusting

- Grease a baking dish then arrange the cherries in a single layer in the bottom.

- Beat together the flour, sugar, eggs, and milk to make a smooth batter.

- Pour the batter over the cherries and bake in a preheated oven, at 350°F, for 25 minutes, until golden and just set. Serve warm with a dusting of confectioners' sugar.

10 Fried Cherry Sandwiches

For each sandwich, butter 2 slices of bread, spread 1 slice with cherry preserves, and sandwich together. Beat 1 egg in a shallow bowl and dip both sides of the sandwich in it. Heat 2 tablespoons butter in a skillet, add the sandwich, and cook for 2 minutes, until golden. Turn and cook the other side. Serve warm, dusted with confectioners' sugar.

20 Warm Cherry Waffles

Heat ¼ cup granulated sugar, 4 tablespoons butter, and ¼ cup orange juice in a large skillet until the butter has melted and the sugar dissolved. Drain 1 (15 oz) can pitted black cherries, reserving the juice. Mix the cherry juice with 1 tablespoon cornstarch blended to a paste with 1 tablespoon cold water and pour into the pan. Bring to a boil, stirring, until thickened and smooth. Place 4 prepared waffles in the pan with the sauce. Add the cherries and heat through for a few minutes, spooning some of the sauce over the pancakes. Serve with cream.

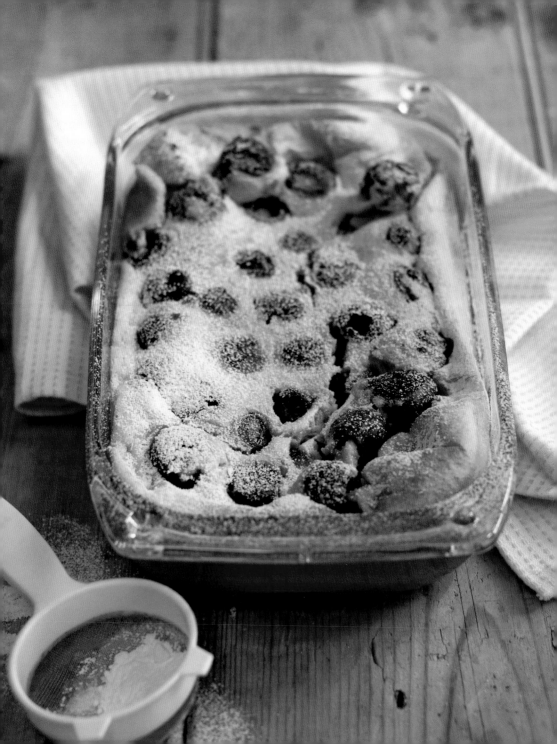

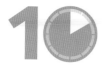 # Chocolate-Dipped Fruits

Makes about 30

6 oz semisweet or milk chocolate, broken into pieces

6 oz white chocolate, broken into pieces

10 strawberries, with stalks on

1 banana, thickly sliced

10 pieces of canned pineapple

- Heat the semisweet or milk and white chocolate in separate heatproof bowls over separate saucepans of simmering water, making sure the bottoms of the bowl don't touch the water. Let heat for a few minutes, stirring occasionally, until the chocolate is melted and smooth. Transfer the melted chocolates to 2 small cups or serving bowls.

- Stick the pieces of fruit onto toothpicks and dip into the warm chocolate. Either eat immediately or place on baking sheets lined with parchment paper and chill for a few minutes, until the chocolate sets.

 ### Iced Berries with Warm Chocolate

Sauce Spread 2 cups frozen mixed berries, such as raspberries, blackberries, and blueberries, over a plate and let defrost slightly for 15 minutes. Meanwhile, put 4 oz semisweet, milk, or white chocolate into a heatproof bowl with ⅔ cup heavy cream. Place the bowl over a saucepan of simmering water and stir until the chocolate has melted and the sauce is smooth. Spoon the semifrozen berries into glasses or dishes and serve with the warm chocolate sauce poured over them.

 ### Warm Chocolate and Berry Tart

Heat 14 oz prepared vanilla pudding with 6 oz semisweet chocolate, broken into pieces, in a saucepan over low heat until the chocolate melts and the pudding is smooth. Cool for 10 minutes, then pour into a prepared pie crust. Chop 2 cups mixed mixed berries and spoon over the pudding. Dust with confectioners' sugar and serve.

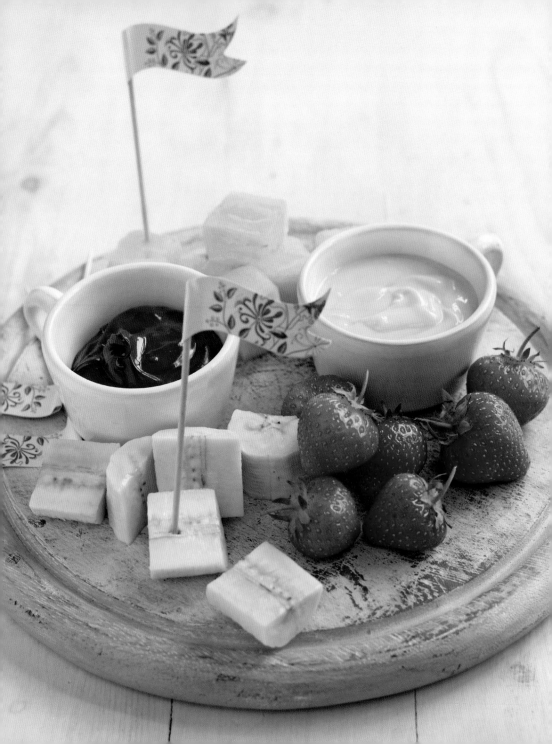

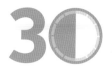

Iced Banana and Raspberry Buns

Makes 12

1 cup all-purpose flour
1 teaspoon baking powder
2 tablespoons granulated sugar
1 ripe banana, mashed
1 egg
4 tablespoons milk
4 tablespoons butter, melted
⅓ cup raspberries
⅓ cup confectioners' sugar
1–2 teaspoons water
pink food coloring
sugar flowers, to decorate

- Line a 12-cup muffin pan with paper cake liners.

- Sift the flour and baking powder into a bowl and stir in the granulated sugar. Mix together the mashed banana, egg, milk, and melted butter in a separate bowl, then add to the dry ingredients. Add the raspberries and stir until mixed.

- Spoon the batter into the cake liners and bake in a preheated oven, at 350°F, for 15 minutes, until golden and just firm to the touch. Let cool slightly.

- Mix the confectioners' sugar with the measured water to make a smooth icing. Add a drop of pink food coloring and stir to mix. Spoon onto the cakes and decorate with sugar flowers.

---

1 Banana and Honey Frosted Cakes

Mix together 1 ripe mashed banana, ¾ cup cream cheese, and 1 tablespoon honey. Spread over the top of store-bought plain cupcakes and top each with a banana chip.

2 Banana and Honey Cakes

Make up 1 (15 oz) package yellow cupcake mix according to the package directions. Mash 1 ripe banana with a fork and stir into the cake mixture with 1 tablespoon honey. Spoon the mixture into paper cake liners and bake in a preheated oven, at 350°F, for 15 minutes. Brush with a little extra honey while warm and stick a banana chip on the top of each cake.

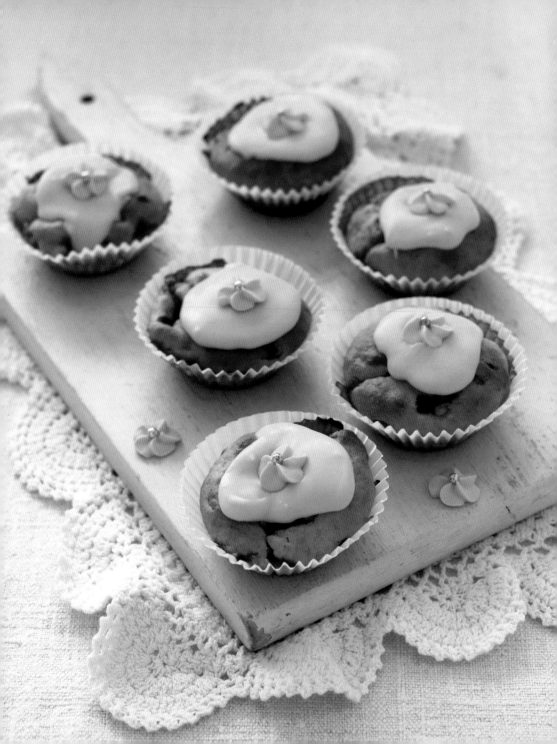

30 Saucy Lemon Desserts

Serves 4

butter, for greasing
1 egg, separated
3 tablespoons granulated sugar
1 tablespoon all-purpose flour
finely grated rind and juice
  of 1 lemon
½ cup milk
confectioners' sugar, for dusting

- Lightly grease 4 ovenproof dishes or tea cups, then stand them in a roasting pan.

- Place the egg yolk and granulated sugar in a large bowl and beat together, using an electric mixer, until creamy. Beat in the flour, lemon rind, and lemon juice until smooth, then gradually beat in the milk.

- In a separate clean bowl, beat the egg white until soft peaks form. Lightly fold into the lemon mixture and spoon into the cups or dishes. Pour boiling water into the roasting pan to come halfway up the sides of the cups or dishes and bake in a preheated oven, at 350°F, for 15–20 minutes, until risen and golden. The sauce will separate during cooking underneath the fluffy tops.

- Dust with confectioners' sugar and serve immediately.

---

1 Pound Cake with Lemon Pudding

Pour 1¾ cups prepared vanilla pudding into a microwave-proof small bowl and heat in the microwave on full power for 3 minutes. Stir in ¼ cup lemon curd and heat for another minute on full power. Cut 4 thick slices of pound cake into chunks, spread out over a microwave-proof plate, and heat on full power for 30 seconds, until warm. Divide the cake among 4 bowls and pour the warm pudding over the cake.

2 Sponge Cake with Lemon Sauce

Using an electric mixer, beat together ½ cup packed sunflower spread, ⅔ cup granulated sugar, 1 cup all-purpose flour, 1 teaspoon baking powder, and 2 eggs until soft and creamy. Spoon the batter into a medium microwave-proof baking dish and cook in the microwave on full power for 3 minutes, turning once. Let stand for 1 minute. Heat ¼ cup lemon curd in the microwave for 30 seconds, until warmed. Spoon the curd over the sponge cake and serve with whipped cream.

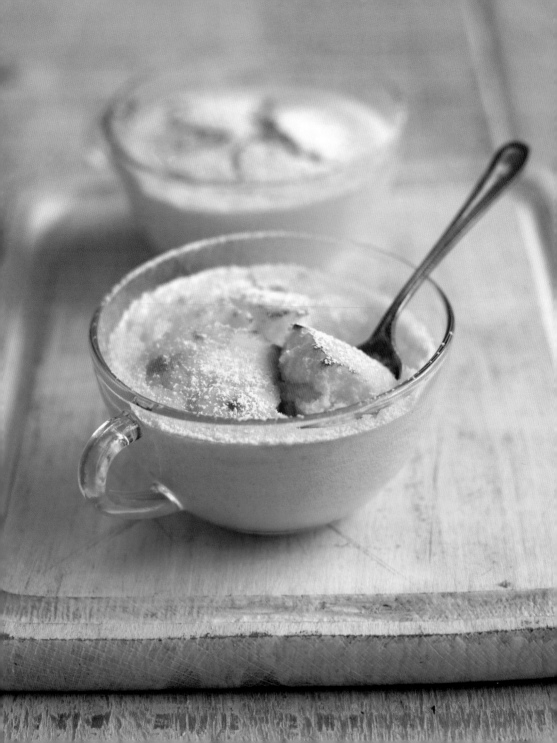

30 Chocolate Oat Bars

Makes 10

1½ sticks butter, plus extra
   for greasing
1½ tablespoons light corn syrup
¾ cup firmly packed light
   brown sugar
3 cups rolled oats
3 tablespoons good-quality
   cocoa powder

- Grease a shallow 8 inch square baking pan.

- Melt the butter, corn syrup, and sugar in a saucepan over low heat until just melted but not boiling. Remove from the heat and stir in the oats and cocoa powder.

- Press the batter into the prepared pan and bake in a preheated oven, at 300°F, for 20 minutes.

- Let cool slightly, then cut into rectangles.

 Crunchy Chocolate Oat Crisp

Melt 3 tablespoons sunflower spread in a saucepan. Remove from the heat and stir in 2 tablespoons demerara sugar or raw sugar and ½ cup rolled oats. Spread out over an aluminum foil-lined baking sheet and cook under a preheated hot broiler for 2–3 minutes, stirring occasionally, until golden and crisp. Transfer to a bowl and stir in ¼ cup chocolate chips. Sprinkle the mixture over sliced bananas or yogurt.

 Mini Chocolate Oat Bites

Place ½ cup packed sunflower spread in a microwave-proof bowl with ¼ cup firmly packed light brown sugar and 2 tablespoons honey. Heat in the microwave on full power for 30 seconds, until just melted. Stir in 1⅓ cups rolled oats, 1 cup all-purpose flour, 1 teaspoon baking powder, ½ teaspoon ground allspice, and ¼ cup chocolate chips. Place about 30 heaping teaspoons of the batter on 2 baking sheets lined with parchment paper and bake in a preheated oven, at 350°F, for 10 minutes, until golden. Eat warm or cold.

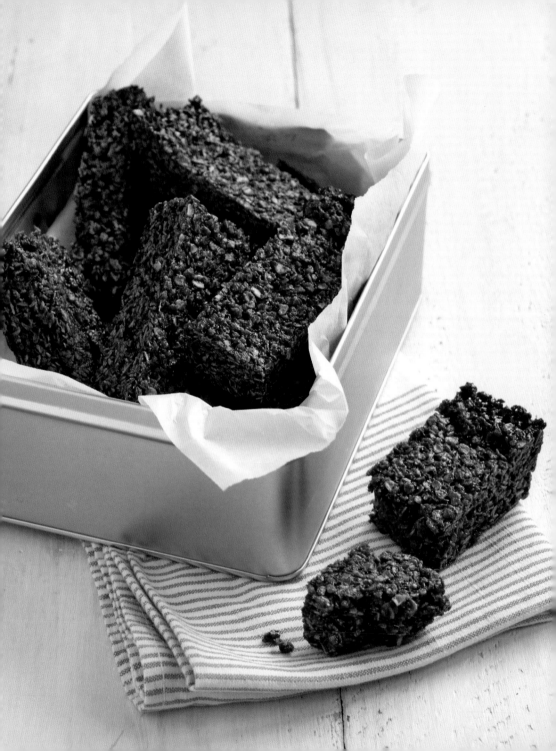

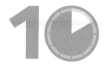 # Quick Mixed Berry Ice Cream

Serves 4

4 cups frozen mixed berries
⅓ cup confectioners' sugar
1 tablespoon honey
2 cups prepared vanilla pudding
sugar sprinkles, to decorate

- Reserve a few of the fruits for decoration. Place the remaining fruits in a food processor with the confectioners' sugar and honey and blend until smooth.

- While the motor is running, slowly pour in the vanilla pudding until the mixture is thick and forms a soft ice cream.

- Spoon into paper cups or bowls, then decorate with sugar sprinkles before serving.

---

2 Ice Cream Meringues with Mixed Berry Sauce

Place 4 cups frozen mixed berries in a saucepan with ⅓ cup confectioners' sugar. Heat, stirring, until the fruits are defrosted. Blend the fruits and their juice in a food processor until smooth. Add a little water if the mixture is too thick and blend again until smooth. Place scoops of ice cream on prepared meringue nests and serve with the fruit sauce.

3 Iced Mixed berry Meringue Bombes

Blend 4 cups frozen mixed berries in a food processor with ⅓ cup confectioners' sugar and 1¼ cups prepared vanilla pudding. Transfer to a bowl and quickly stir in 3 crushed meringue nests. Spoon the mixture into 6 plastic wrap-lined individual bowls or ramekins. Freeze for 20 minutes, then turn out, remove the plastic wrap, and serve with raspberries.

KID-TAST-XYE

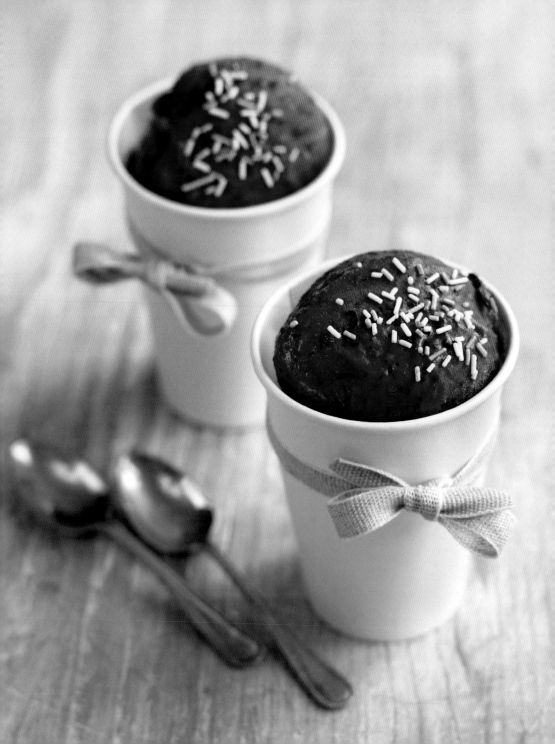

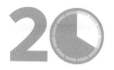

20 Spiced Raisin and Cranberry Cookies

Makes 8

1 stick butter

⅔ cup firmly packed
light brown sugar

1 tablespoon light corn syrup

1 cup all-purpose flour

1 teaspoon baking powder

½ teaspoon ground allspice

1⅓ cups rolled oats

⅓ cup raisins

⅓ cup dried cranberries

- Line 2 baking sheets with parchment paper.

- Heat the butter, sugar, and corn syrup in a saucepan until just melted. Remove from the pan and stir in the flour, baking powder, allspice, oats, and fruit.

- Roll the mixture into 8 balls, place on the prepared baking sheets, and flatten slightly. Bake in a preheated oven, at 350°F, for 10–12 minutes.

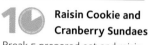

Raisin Cookie and Cranberry Sundaes Break 5 prepared oat and raisin cookies into pieces and sprinkle them over scoops of soft vanilla ice cream in glasses. Top with a sprinkling of dried cranberries.

Spiced Cranberry and Raisin Cupcakes In a food processor, blend 1 cup all-purpose flour, 1 teaspoon baking powder, ½ teaspoon ground allspice, ½ cup sunflower spread, ⅔ cup granulated sugar, and 2 eggs until smooth and creamy. Stir in 1 finely chopped Pippin apple, ½ cup raisins, and 3 tablespoons dried cranberries. Spoon into 12 paper cake liners and bake in a preheated oven, at 350°F, for 15–20 minutes.

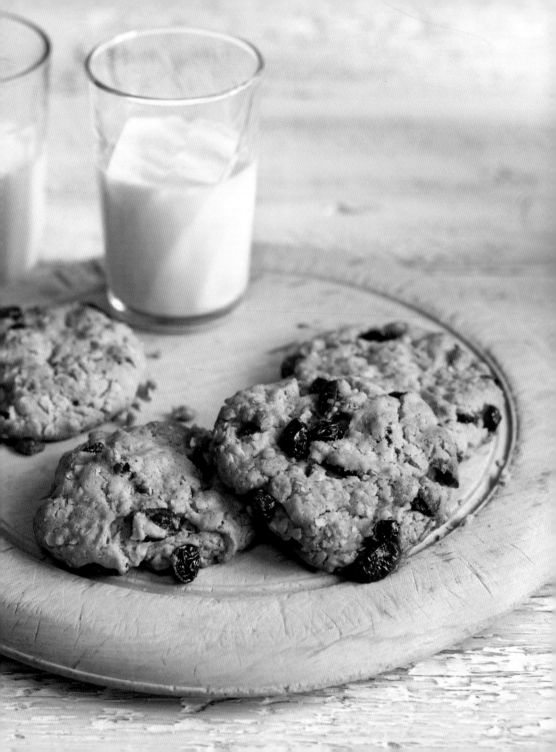

30 Wheat-Free Gooey Chocolate Brownies

Makes 16

8 oz semisweet chocolate, broken into pieces

1 stick unsalted butter, softened

1¼ cups firmly packed light brown sugar

4 eggs, beaten

1 teaspoon vanilla extract

½ cup ground almonds (almond meal)

½ cup cocoa powder

- Line a shallow 6 inch square cake pan with parchment paper.

- Heat the chocolate and butter in a heatproof bowl over a saucepan of simmering water, making sure the bottom of the bowl doesn't touch the water, until melted and smooth. Remove from the heat and cool slightly.

- Add the sugar and beat together until fluffy. Gradually beat in the eggs, vanilla extract, and melted chocolate. Add the ground almonds, sift in the cocoa powder, and stir well to mix.

- Spoon the mixture into the prepared pan and bake in a preheated oven, at 350°F, for 20 minutes, until just firm to the touch but still a little soft. Let cool slightly before cutting into 16 squares.

1 Wheat-Free Brownies with Warm Chocolate Fudge Sauce

In a small saucepan gently heat ¼ cup firmly packed light brown sugar, 4 tablespoons butter, ⅓ cup heavy cream, and 4 oz semisweet chocolate, broken into pieces. Stir occasionally until the chocolate has melted, the sugar has dissolved, and the sauce is smooth. Pour the sauce over prepared wheat-free brownies (see above) and serve with a scoop of ice cream.

2 Wheat-Free Mars Bar Krispie Bites

Chop 2 Mars Bars and place in a heatproof bowl with 4 tablespoons butter over a saucepan of simmering water. Stir occasionally until the mixture is melted and smooth. Remove from the heat and stir in 1¾ cups Rice Krispies or similar cereal, until evenly coated. Place spoonfuls of the mixture on a baking sheet lined with parchment paper and chill in the freezer for 10 minutes to set.

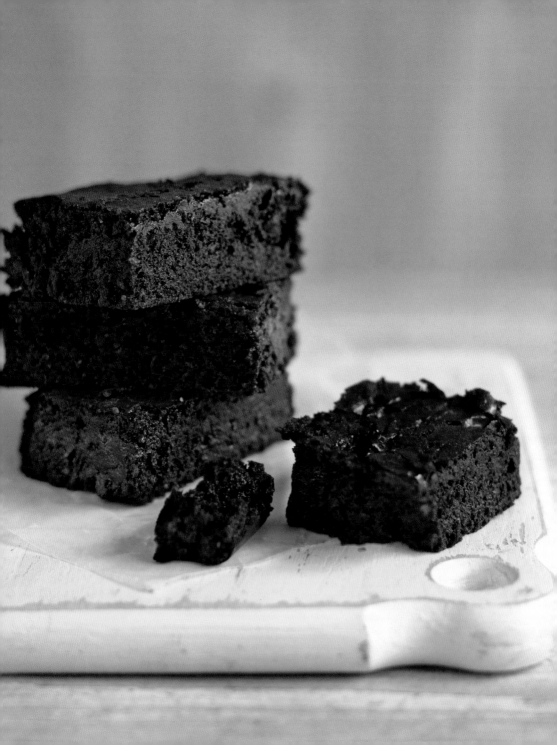

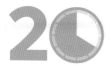

Chocolate Muffin Trifles

Serves 4

1¼ cups prepared vanilla pudding

4 oz milk chocolate, broken into pieces

2 chocolate muffins, broken into chunks

1 (15 oz) can black cherry pie filling

⅔ cup whipping cream

crumbled chocolate or chocolate shavings, to decorate

- Heat the vanilla pudding and chocolate in a small saucepan over low heat, stirring, until the chocolate melts and the pudding is smooth. Let cool slightly.

- Divide the muffins among 4 glasses or bowls, or 1 large bowl, and spoon the cherry pie filling over the top.

- Pour the chocolate pudding over the cherry filling. Whip the cream until just thick enough to form soft peaks, then place spoonfuls on the pudding. Sprinkle the crumbled or shaved chocolate over the top.

 Chocolate Muffin and Sundae

Chop 2 chocolate muffins into chunks and divide among 4 sundae glasses. Add 2 scoops of vanilla ice cream and a sprinkling of jelly beans to each. Pour 1½ cups prepared chocolate pudding over the top and finish off with a spoonful of whipped cream and a few jelly beans.

 Baked Chocolate Croissant Pudding

Split 4 prepared croissants in half, spread with 3 tablespoons chocolate hazelnut spread, and sandwich back together again. Cut each croissant into 3 pieces and place in a shallow ovenproof dish. Lightly beat 2 eggs with 1¼ cups chocolate milkshake and pour the mixture over the croissants. Bake in a preheated oven, at 350°F, for 20 minutes, until the custard has softly set. Serve warm.

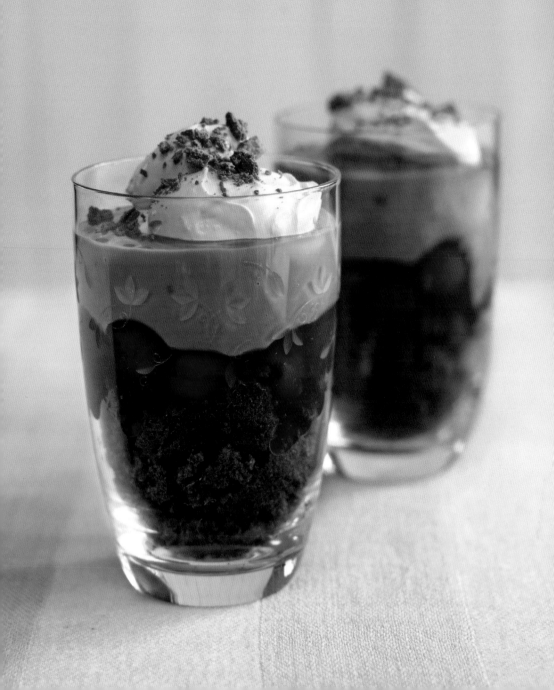

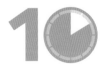

Slippery Snake

Serves 8

1 (5 oz) can chunk light tuna in water, drained
½ cup cream cheese
1 (8¾ oz) can corn kernels, drained
4 bagels, halved
8 cherry tomatoes, halved
1 black grape, halved
1 strip of cucumber skin, cut into a forked tongue

- Mix together the tuna, cream cheese, and corn.

- Cut each bagel half in half again to make 8 semicircles and arrange them end to end on a board to resemble a curly snake.

- Spread the tuna mixture on the bagels and arrange the cherry tomatoes, cut side down, along the length. Place the grape halves at one end for eyes, and finish with the cucumber forked tongue.

 Dough Ball Caterpillar

Cook 12 garlic butter dough balls in a preheated oven according to the package directions. Arrange in a wiggly line on a bed of micro salad greens. To make ladybuds, place halved plum tomatoes, cut side down, then top with small pieces of black olive stuck on with a little mayonnaise for the spots and eyes.

Burger Bugs

Cook 8 burgers under a preheated medium broiler according to the package directions. Cut 8 burger buns in half and, using scissors, snip the top half of the buns into a zigzag shape to look like teeth. Place the burgers in the buns with lettuce. Arrange 2 halves of a cucumber slice poking out from underneath for feet, then stick 2 cherry tomatoes on toothpicks toward the front of the top of the bun to look like "googly" eyes.

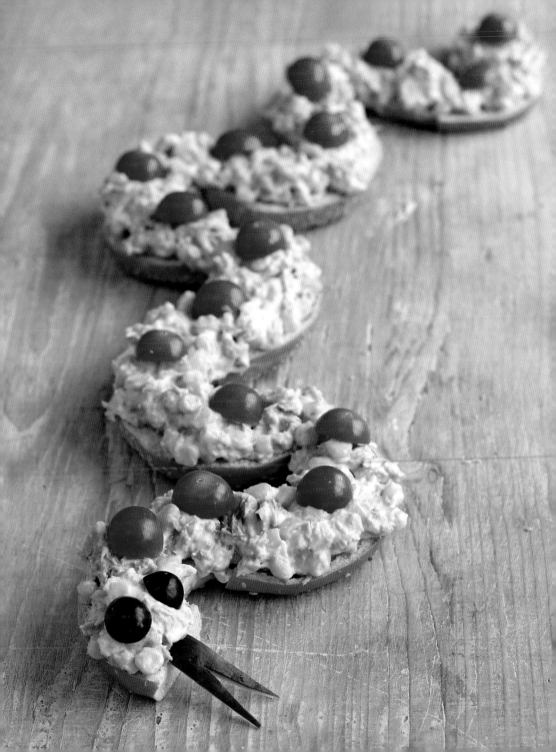

30 Pizza Faces

Makes 4

4 mini pizza crusts
1¼ cups prepared pizza sauce
8 thin slices of salami or
  pepperoni
½ cup shredded
  mozzarella cheese
4 pitted ripe black olives, halved
2 cherry tomatoes, halved
4 small strips of green bell pepper
8 strips of red bell pepper

- Place the pizza crusts on a baking sheet and spread the pizza topping over each one, leaving a small border around the edge.

- Place 2 slices of salami or pepperoni on each pizza for eyes, sprinkle with a little mozzarella, and place a black olive half in the center of each one. Add half a cherry tomato for the nose and a strip of green bell pepper for the mouth.

- Place the red bell pepper slices at the top for ears, then sprinkle with the remaining mozzarella for hair.

- Bake in a preheated oven, at 400°F, for 10–15 minutes, until golden. Serve warm.

10 Pizza Muffin Faces

Cut 4 English muffins in half and toast both sides. Spread each cut side with a generous teaspoonful of pizza sauce, then sprinkle with some shredded mozzarella cheese. Broil until golden and arrange cucumber slices, cherry tomatoes, and salad greens to look like faces and hair.

20 Funny Face Cheese Pizzas

Place a sprinkling of drained canned corn kernels to look like hair on 4 prepared cheese pizzas. Arrange pitted olives for eyes, cherry tomato halves for noses, and a strip of salami for a mouth. Place the pizzas on baking sheets and bake in a preheated oven, at 400°F, for 10 minutes or according to the package directions.

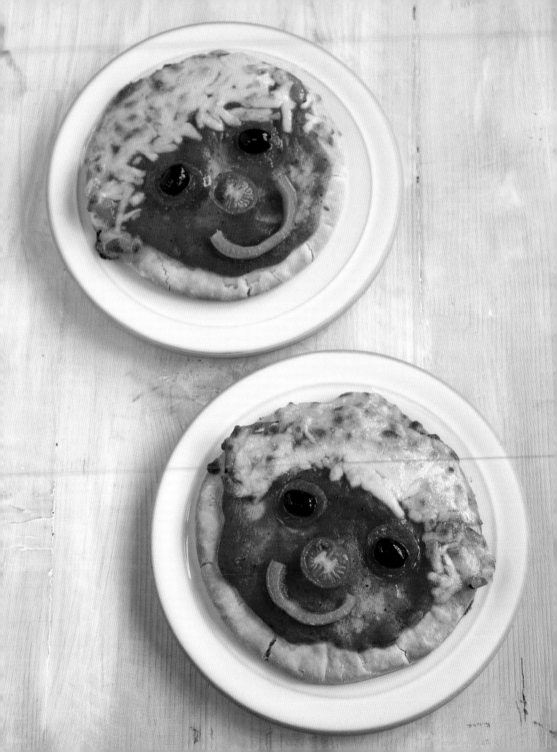

30 Chocolate and Cranberry Crunch Squares

Makes 9

1 stick butter
¼ cup granulated sugar
1 tablespoon light corn syrup
4 teaspoons cocoa powder
2 cups crushed graham crackers
½ cup cranberries

For the topping

4 oz milk chocolate,
   broken into pieces
1 tablespoon butter
colorful candy-coated chocolates,
   to decorate

- Line a shallow 7 inch square pan with plastic wrap.

- Melt the butter, sugar, corn syrup, and cocoa powder in a saucepan, stirring until smooth. Remove from the heat and stir in the crushed crackers and cranberries.

- Spoon the batter into the prepared pan. Press it down firmly and evenly with the back of a spoon. Place in the freezer for 5 minutes to chill.

- To make the topping, heat the chocolate and butter in a heatproof bowl over a saucepan of simmering water, making sure the bottom of the bowl doesn't touch the water, until melted and smooth.

- Pour the chocolate topping over the cookie crust and spread evenly. Decorate with colorful candies, then return to the freezer for 10 minutes to set. Cut into squares to serve.

---

10 Rainbow Cookies Spread plain cookies with chocolate hazelnut spread from a jar and sprinkle with cake-decorating confetti dots or mini colorful candy-coated chocolates.

20 Chocolate and Cranberry Krispie Cakes Heat 8 oz semisweet chocolate, broken into pieces, with ¼ cup light corn syrup and 4 tablespoons butter in a large heatproof bowl over a saucepan of simmering water, stirring occasionally, until melted and smooth. Stir in 3 cups Rice Krispies or similar cereal, 3 tablespoons dried cranberries, and ½ (4 oz) package slivered dried strawberries. Spoon into paper cake liners and place in the freezer for 5 minutes to set.

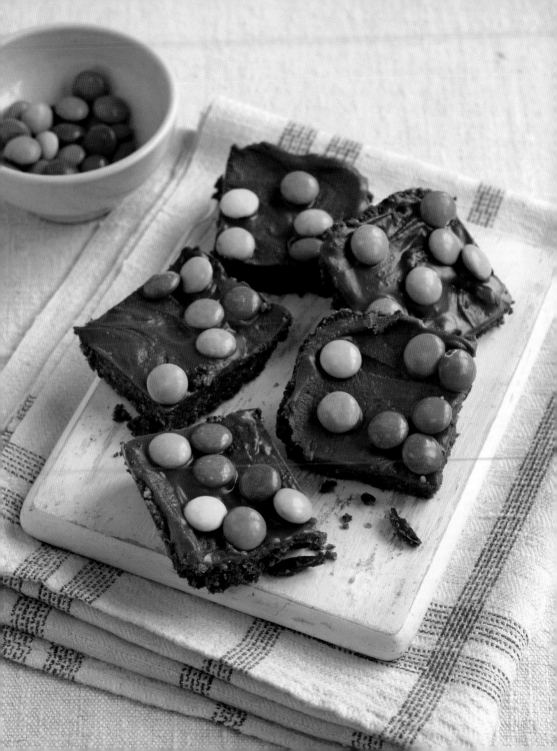

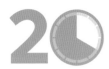 # Pirate and Princess Cakes

Makes 12

12 prepared plain cupcakes
1 (12 oz) container prepared
  vanilla frosting

For the pirates

2 oz red ready-to-use
  rolled fondant
tubes of white and black
  writing icing

For the princesses

mixture of colored candies,
  such as gumdrops, jelly
  candies, licorice pieces, mini
  marshmallows, and cake
  decoration sprinkles
silver ball cake decorations
edible glitter dust (optional)

- For the pirate cakes, spread 6 cakes with vanilla frosting and level the surface. Roll out the red fondant, cut 6 semicircles to fit the top third of each cake, and place on the cakes to make the scarf hats. Roll any scraps into little logs and twists and stick on one side of the hats as knots. Squeeze little dots over the hats, or crossbone shapes, with the white writing icing. Use the black writing icing to make a dot for one eye, an eye patch for the other, a dot for the nose, and a large semicircle for the mouth.

- For the Princess cakes, swirl a generous spoonful of vanilla frosting on the top of the 6 remaining cakes. Pile the candies on top with a few silver balls, then sprinkle with edible glitter dust, if using.

 ### Buried Treasure Cakes

Spread 12 prepared plain cupcakes with 1 (12 oz) container prepared vanilla frosting. Put 3 oz boiled fruit-flavored candies in a plastic food bag and crush them with a rolling pin. Stick them into the frosting with a few silver ball cake decorations.

 ### Treasure Island and Fairy-Tale Castle Cakes

Divide 6 oz white ready-to-use rolled fondant in half and knead pink food coloring into one half and green into the other. Roll out the fondants and cut 6 circles from each, large enough to cover the tops of 12 prepared plain cupcakes. Mix 2 tablespoons confectioners' sugar with a little water to make a smooth icing, spread a little over the top of each cake, and stick the rolled-out fondant circles on the top. For the fairy-tale castles, arrange miniature marshmallows in a square on the top of each cake, securing with a dab of pink icing. Stick a flag (pink paper stuck on a toothpick) in the center. For the treasure island cakes, sprinkle crushed graham crackers around the edge of the green icing for sand. Make palm trees from thin chocolate cookies and leftover green fondant, rolled and snipped for the leaves. Push down into the center of each cake.

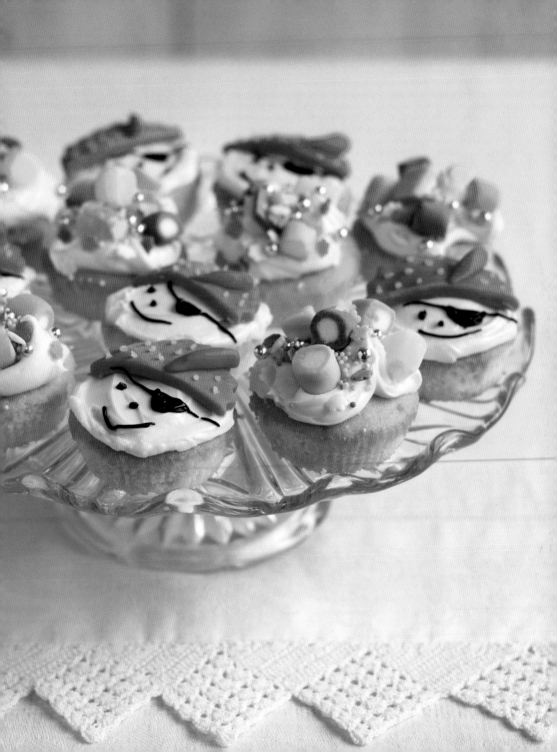

3⊙ Gingerbread People Beach Party

Makes 6

2 oz pink ready-to-use
rolled fondant

2 oz blue ready-to-use
rolled fondant

6 prepared plain gingerbread
people

writing icing tubes in red, black,
and yellow

⅔ cup demerara sugar or
other raw sugar

paper cocktail umbrellas

- Roll out the pink and blue fondants and cut out bikini shapes for 3 of the gingerbread people and shorts for the other 3. Stick in place with a little of the writing icing. Pipe on faces and hair with the writing icing tubes.

- With the ready-to-use rolled fondant scraps, reroll and cut out beach towels, flip flops, beach balls, books, etc.

- Spread the demerara sugar out on a board to make the sand, then arrange the gingerbread people with their towels and accessories and the cocktail umbrellas to make a beach party.

 Bow Ties and Hearts Gingerbread Men Roll out 2 oz red ready-to-use rolled fondant and cut out 3 hearts large enough to cover the body of 3 prepared gingerbread men, and 3 large bow ties. Stick onto 6 gingerbread men using a tube of white writing icing and decorate with silver ball cake decorations. Pipe faces with the tube of icing.

 Chocolate-Dipped Gingerbread Men Heat 4 oz milk chocolate in a heatproof bowl over a saucepan of simmering water, making sure the bottom of the bowl doesn't touch the water, until melted and smooth. Dip the top of the heads and the toes of 6 prepared gingerbread men into the chocolate and place on a baking sheet lined with parchment paper. Place in the refrigerator for 5 minutes to set. Using a tube of white writing icing, pipe dots for eyes and a nose and a smiling mouth. Stick colorful candy-coated chocolates or gumdrops down the center for buttons.

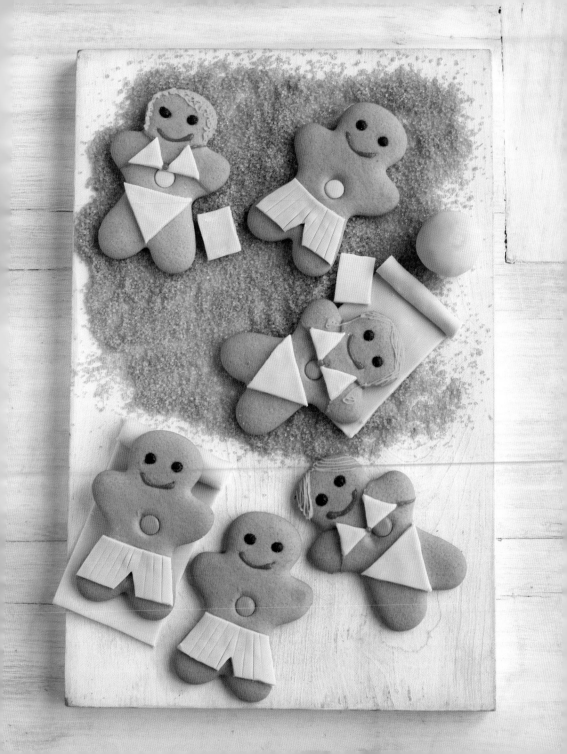

10 Mocktails

Each mocktail serves 2

Fizzy Fish
6 fizzy fish jelly candies
⅔ cup mango juice
chilled lemon-flavored soda

Paradise Cooler
1¼ cups pineapple juice
2 scoops of vanilla ice cream

Beach Babes
⅔ cup orange juice
⅔ cup cranberry juice drink
sparkling mineral water
2 orange slices, to decorate
2 strawberries, to decorate

- For the Fizzy Fish, place the candies in the bottom of 2 glasses. Add the mango juice and top up with lemon-flavored soda. Serve with toothpicks to see who can "fish" out the candies first before drinking the beverage.

- For the Paradise Cooler, pour the pineapple juice into 2 glasses and top each with a scoop of ice cream. Decorate with cocktail umbrellas and long spoons to eat the ice cream.

- For the Beach Babes, divide the juices between 2 glasses, top up with sparkling water, and decorate the rim of the each glass with an orange slice and a strawberry.

20 Swampy Punch

Put 10 grapes in the freezer for 15 minutes to chill. In a small bowl, mix together ¼ cup strawberry syrup and 2½ cups cola. Add 4 scoops of chocolate ice cream and some jelly worms and other jelly shapes. Add the semifrozen grapes just before serving. Pour into glasses—but make sure the decorations and grapes are removed and eatened before the child drinks the cola.

30 Mixed Berry and Apple Smoothies with Vegetable Chips

Using a vegetable peeler, cut 1 parsnip, 1 carrot, and 1 sweet potato into thin ribbons. Dry on paper towels, then place in a bowl with 2 tablespoons olive oil. Season with salt and black pepper and mix well to coat. Spread the slices out over a large baking sheet and cook in a preheated oven, at 425°F, for about 5 minutes, until golden and crisp. To make the smoothie, blend 2 cups hulled strawberries, 1½ cups frozen raspberries, and 3 peeled, cored, and quartered Pippin apples in a food processor until smooth. Add 1¼ cups orange juice and blend again. Pour into glasses and place a strawberry on the rim of each glass. Serve with the vegetable chips.

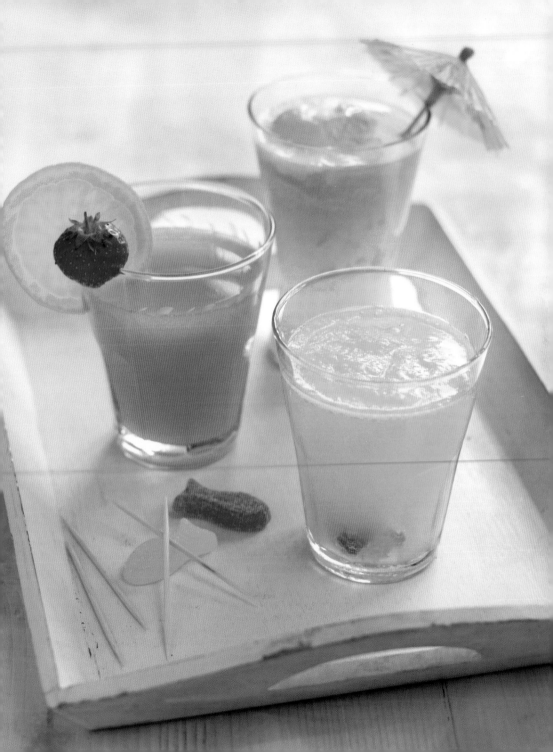

1⬤ Magic Wands

Makes 10

3 oz white chocolate, broken
  into pieces
10 breadsticks
colorful cake decoration sprinkles

- Put a baking sheet lined with parchment paper into the freezer to chill.

- Heat the chocolate in a heatproof bowl over a saucepan of simmering water, making sure the bottom of the bowl doesn't touch the water, until melted and smooth. Pour into a mug (this gives more depth of chocolate for dipping).

- Dip one end of each breadstick into the chocolate and shake off any excess. Roll in the sprinkles and place on the cold baking sheet. Return to the freezer for a few minutes to set.

2⬤ **Glitter Stars**
Unroll 1 sheet store-bought rolled dough pie crust and cut out star shapes using a 3 inch cutter. Place on a baking sheet and bake in a preheated oven, at 375°F, for 10 minutes, until golden and crisp. Mix 1 cup confectioners' sugar with about 2 teaspoons water to make a smooth icing. Drizzle it over the cookies and sprinkle with colorful cake decoration sprinkles and a dusting of edible glitter.

3⬤ **Yum Yum Twists**
Unroll 1 (8 oz) can crescent roll dough. Cut the dough into 12 strips widthwise. Twist 2 strips together, securing the ends with a dab of water, then place on a baking sheet. Repeat to make 6 twists. Brush with a little milk and bake in a preheated oven, at 400°F, for about 10 minutes, until golden. Mix 1 cup confectioners' sugar with about 1 tablespoon water to make a smooth, runny icing.

Drizzle over the yum yums and sprinkle with colorful cake decoration sprinkles.

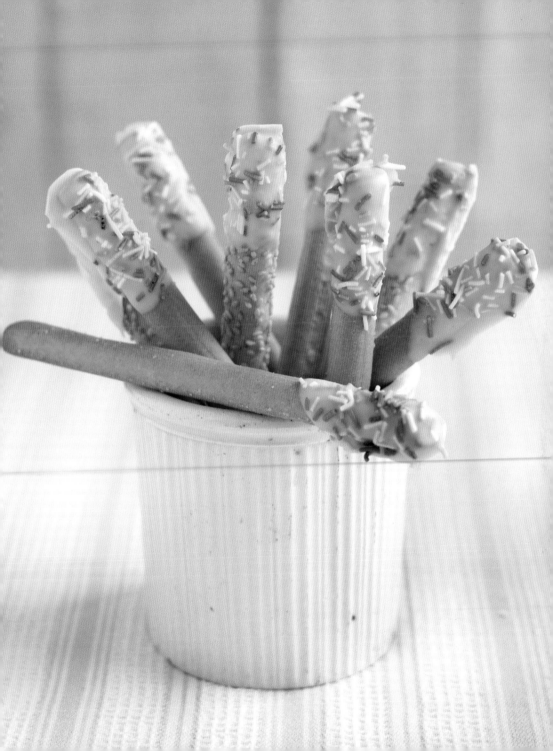

2 Number Cookies

Makes about 10

1 sheet store-bought rolled dough
  pie crust
¼ cup strawberry preserves
confectioners' sugar, for dusting

- Unroll the dough and cut out letters using large cookie cutters to spell children's names, "Happy Birthday," or any other message of your choice, cutting each letter twice.

- Place on baking sheets and bake in a preheated oven, at 375°F, for 10 minutes, until golden and crisp.

- Place the letters together in pairs. Spread one with a layer of preserves and top with the other. Dust with confectioners' sugar and arrange the cookies to spell out names or your chosen message.

1 Message Cookies

Arrange colorful candies on prepared chocolate cookies to form a letter on each cookie. Stick in place with a dab of icing from a tube of writing icing. Arrange the cookies to spell out your chosen name or message.

3 Lollipop Cookies

Unroll 1 sheet store-bought rolled dough pie crust and cut out 12 circles, using a 3 inch cutter. Place on 2 baking sheets and carefully push a lollipop or ice cream stick into the side of each circle to reach the center. Bake in a preheated oven, at 375°F, for 10 minutes, until golden. While the cookies are cooking, roll out 4 oz pink or blue ready-to-use rolled fondant and cut out numbers or letters, using cookie cutters. Stick the numbers or letters onto the cookies with a dab of icing from a tube of writing icing and decorate with colorful candies.

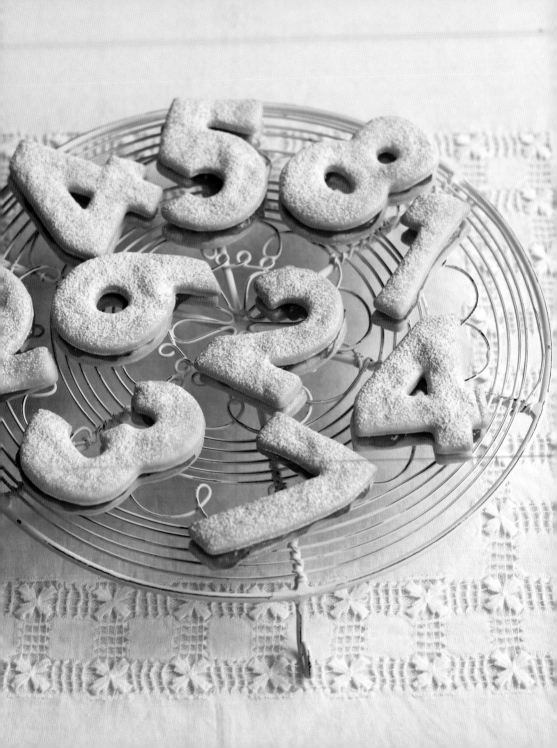

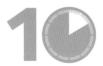 # Cheesy Garlic Bread

Serves 8

1 loaf French bread

½ cup packed prepared garlic and herb butter

1⅓ cups shredded mozzarella cheese

- Cut the French bread in half lengthwise. Spread the garlic and herb butter generously over both halves and place on a baking sheet (cut the bread in half if it is too long for the oven).

- Sprinkle with the mozzarella and bake in a preheated oven, at 425°F, for 5 minutes, until the cheese has melted. Cut into pieces to serve.

 Garlic and Herb Flatbread with Cheese Dip Melt 4 tablespoons butter in a saucepan or in the microwave with 1 crushed garlic clove. Remove from the heat and stir in 1 tablespoon chopped parsley. Brush the mixture over a prepared pizza crust and bake in a preheated oven, at 400°F, for 10 minutes, until crisp and golden. Cut into wedges and serve with a dip made from ½ cup garlic and herb cream cheese beaten with 2 tablespoons milk.

 Cheesy Garlic Ciabatta Beat 1 stick softened butter with 2 crushed garlic cloves and 2 tablespoons chopped parsley. Season with salt and black pepper. Cut a ciabatta loaf into ½ inch slices, but don't cut all the way through. Spread the butter on both sides of each slice. Cut 5 oz mozzarella cheese into slices and insert a piece of cheese between each slice of bread. Wrap the loaf in aluminum foil and cook in a preheated oven, at 400°F, for 15 minutes, until hot and crispy and the cheese has melted. Unwrap, cut through the slices, and serve warm while the cheese is still gooey.

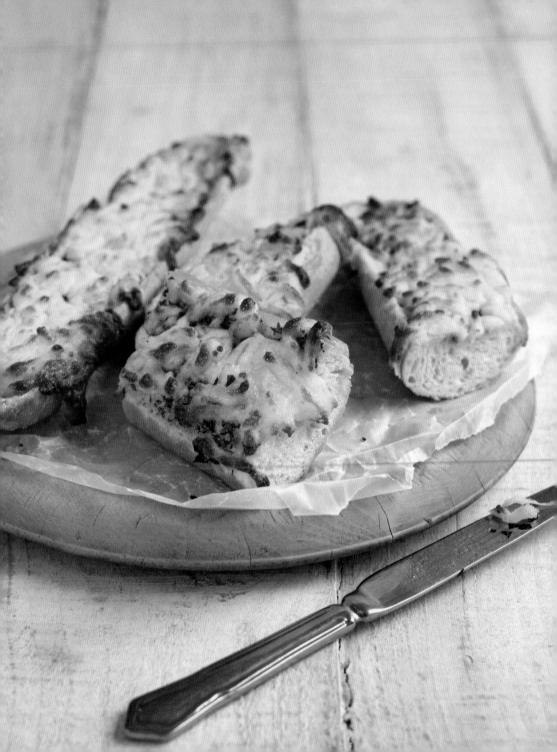

30 Whirly Sausage Rolls

Makes 12

1 sheet ready-to-bake
  puff pastry
16 Vienna sausages or other
  small sausages
beaten egg, to glaze
1 tablespoon sesame seeds
ketchup, to serve

- Unroll the pastry and cut into twelve ¾ inch strips widthwise.

- Wind a strip of pastry around each sausage and place on a baking sheet. Brush with beaten egg and sprinkle with a few sesame seeds.

- Bake in a preheated oven, at 400°F, for 20 minutes, until the pastry is well risen and golden and the sausages are cooked. Serve warm with ketchup for dipping.

10 Barbecue Sausage Wraps Cook

12 Vienna or other small sausages under a preheated broiler for 5 minutes, turning occasionally, until almost cooked. Brush with 2 tablespoons barbecue sauce and cook for 2–3 minutes, until sticky and beginning to char. Warm 6 flour tortillas in the microwave according to the package directions. Place 2 sausages on each, together with some crisp lettuce and a sprinkling of corn kernels. Roll up the wraps to enclose the filling and serve in paper napkins.

20 Cheese and Bacon Hot Dogs

Cook 6 frankfurters under a preheated broiler for 10 minutes, turning occasionally, until cooked through. Using tongs to hold them, carefully cut a slit along the length of each frankfurter. Cut 3 cheese slices each into 4 strips and place 2 strips in the slit in each frankfurter. Wrap a bacon slice around each frankfurter and broil for 5 minutes, until the bacon is cooked. Serve in hot dog rolls with ketchup.

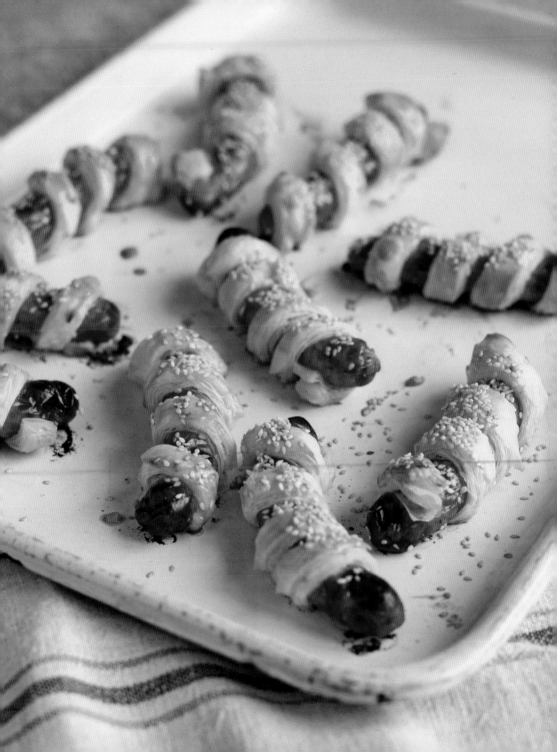

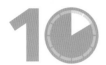 # Rocky Road Popcorn

Serves 4

2 tablespoons sunflower oil

⅔ cup popping corn

6 tablespoons butter

¼ cup instant hot cocoa mix

1¼ cups miniature marshmallows

- Put the oil and popping corn into a large saucepan. Cover with a tight-fitting lid and place the pan over medium heat. Let heat for 2–3 minutes, until you hear the first pop. Shake the pan firmly, keeping the lid in place and the pan on the heat.

- When the popping stops, remove from the heat and transfer the popcorn to a bowl. Add the butter to the pan with the cocoa mix and heat to melt. Pour over the popcorn and stir well.

- Add the marshmallows and serve in paper cones or cups.

 Popcorn Necklaces

Cook 1 (10 oz) microwave butter popcorn according to the package directions. Transfer to a bowl. Thread the popcorn, together with seedless grapes and mini marshmallows, onto lengths of thread, using a blunt tapestry needle. Tie the ends of the thread in a knot to secure.

 Malted Popcorn Balls

Heat 2 tablespoons vegetable oil in a large saucepan with ⅔ cup popping corn. Cover with a tight-fitting lid and cook, shaking the pan occasionally, until the popping stops. Transfer the popcorn into a bowl. Melt 1 stick butter in the hot pan with ¾ cup granulated sugar and 1 tablespoon light corn syrup. Bring to a boil and simmer for about 5 minutes, until golden. Pour the syrup over the popcorn, mix well, and stir in 3 oz coarsely chopped malted milk balls. Shape into balls and place on a baking sheet lined with parchment paper. Chill in the freezer for 10 minutes.

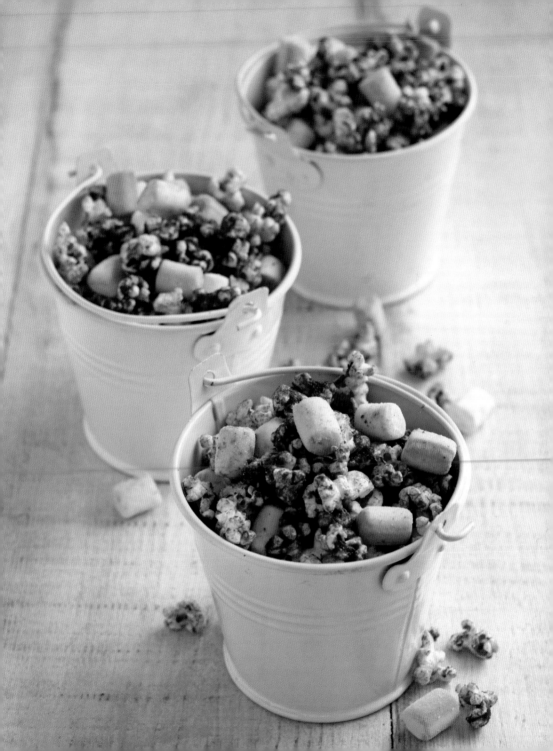

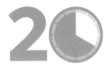

Flower Sandwiches

Serves 8

a drizzle of Worcestershire sauce
or 2 teaspoons yeast extract
1 cup cream cheese
8 slices white bread
8 slices whole-wheat bread
2 cherry tomatoes, halved
2 green grapes, halved
micro greens or lettuce,
to decorate
1 large carrot, peeled and sliced

- Mix together the Worcestershire sauce and cream cheese in a bowl, then spread over the white bread. Cover with the whole-wheat bread and press together firmly. Using a medium-size cutter, cut out as many flower shapes as you can.

- Cut a small circle out of the center of each sandwich, using an apple corer, and stick either a cherry tomato half or grape half in the middle.

- Arrange on a plate or board on a bed of micro greens or lettuce Cut small flower shapes from the carrot slices, using a small cutter and sprinkle over the "grass."

Ham Sticks

Thinly spread a little yeast extract down one side of 12 breadsticks. Cut 6 slices of wafer-thin ham into strips and wrap around the breadsticks, pressing onto the yeast to help it stick. Serve with a selection of raw vegetables, such as carrots, snow peas, and celery.

Party Whirls

Unroll 1 sheet ready-to-bake puff pastry and drizzle with Worchestershipre sauce or spread with yeast extract. Sprinkle with 1 cup shredded cheddar cheese and loosely roll up, starting with one long side. Cut into slices, place on 2 baking sheets lined with parchment paper, and bake in a preheated oven, at 400°F, for 15 minutes, until golden.

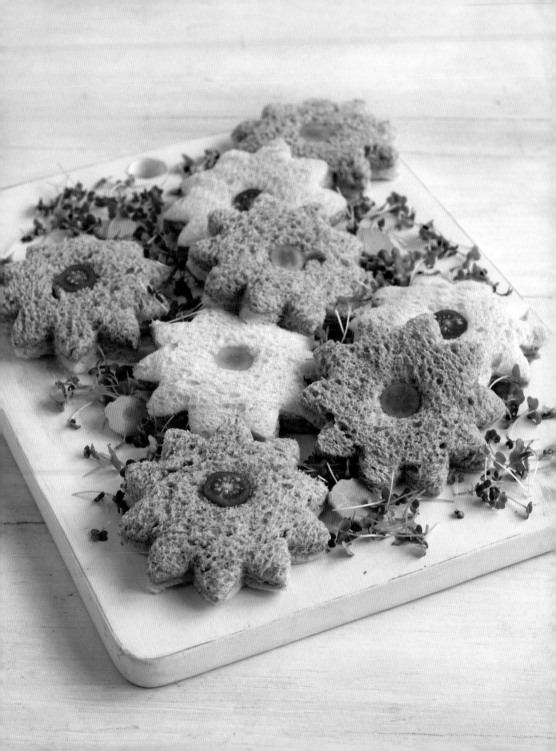

2🕐 BLT Club Sandwiches

Makes 8

4 back bacon slices
6 slices of whole-wheat bread
1 carrot, peeled and grated
½ cup cream cheese
2 tomatoes, sliced
6 lettuce leaves
cherry tomatoes and cucumber
   sticks, to serve

- Cook the bacon under a preheated hot broiler for about 5 minutes, turning once, until crisp.

- Toast the bread slices on both sides.

- Mix together the carrot and cream cheese and spread over 2 slices of the toast. Arrange the tomato slices on top.

- Cover with another slice of toast, and top with the lettuce and bacon. Place the remaining slices of toast on top.

- Press the sandwich stacks down firmly and cut each into 4 triangles. Stick a toothpick flag through each sandwich to hold it all together. Serve with halved cherry tomatoes and cucumber sticks.

1🕐 Sandwich Kebabs

Cut one-quarter of a loaf of French bread into chunks, making sure each piece has some crust on it. Thread onto wooden skewers with cherry tomatoes, cubes of cheese, chunks of cucumber, and cooked Vienna sausages.

3🕐 Surprise Rolls

Cut a slice off the top of 6 round bread rolls and keep the slices for lids. Pull out most of the soft bread from the inside of each roll (this can be saved for making bread crumbs and frozen), leaving a hollow roll. Lightly brush the inside of the rolls with melted butter, then layer up the filling. Between the rolls, divide 4 chopped cooked bacon slices, 2 sliced tomatoes, 4 small lettuce leaves, and ½ cup cream cheese mixed with 1 grated carrot. Press the filling down firmly and replace the lids.

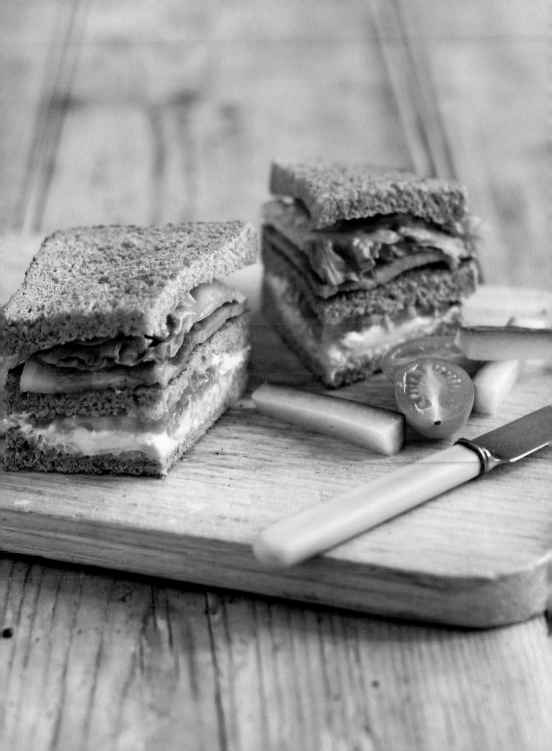

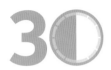

Mini Fish and Chip Cones

Serves 6

2 baking potatoes, scrubbed
¼ cup sunflower oil
1 lb skinless chunky white fish
   fillets, cut into bite-size pieces
2 tablespoons all-purpose flour
1 egg, beaten
1¼ cup dried bread crumbs
salt and black pepper

- Cut the potatoes into thin sticks, coat in 2 tablespoons of the oil, and spread out over a baking sheet. Bake in a preheated oven, at 425°F, for 20 minutes, turning occasionally, until golden and cooked through. Season with salt and black pepper.

- Meanwhile, place the flour on one plate, the beaten egg on another, and the bread crumbs on a third. Dip the fish pieces in the flour, then the egg, and finally the bread crumbs, pressing firmly to coat.

- Heat the remaining oil in a skillet and cook the fish for 5 minutes, turning occasionally, until golden, crisp and cooked through.

- Divide the chips among paper cones made from wax paper and top with the pieces of fish.

Fish Stick Pita Breads Cook 8 fish sticks under a preheated medium broiler for 5–8 minutes, turning occasionally, until golden and cooked through. Cut in half and use to fill warmed pita breads with some lettuce and a spoonful of sour cream and chive dip on each.

Fish and Chip Rolls Place 8 fish sticks and 6 oz prepared thin-cut oven fries on a baking sheet and cook in a preheated oven, at 425°F, for 15 minutes, turning once, until golden and cooked. Split 4 soft white submarine rolls and fill with the fish sticks, fries, a few lettuce leaves and cucumber slices, and a squirt of ketchup.

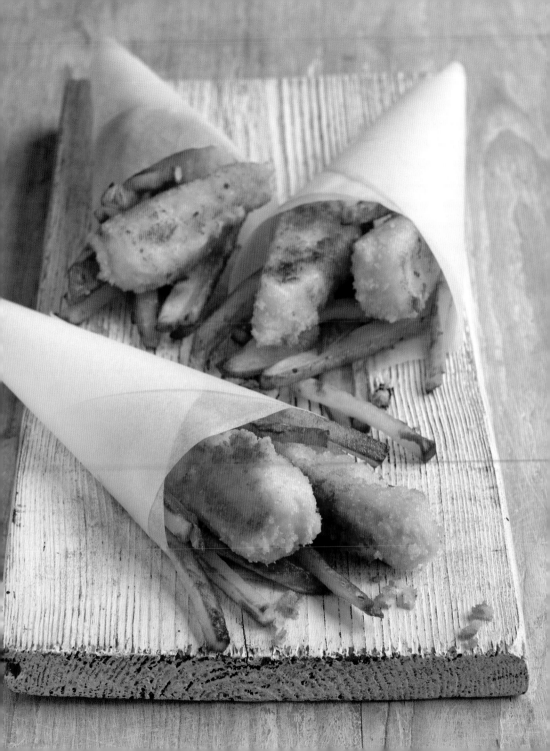

3️⃣ Penny Candy Sheet Cake

Makes 12

¾ cup packed sunflower spread
¾ cup granulated sugar
3 eggs, beaten
1⅓ cups all-purpose flour
1¼ teaspoons baking powder
1 cup confectioners' sugar
1½ tablespoons lemon juice
mixed soft candies, such
   as licorice pieces, gumdrops,
   and jelly candies, to decorate

- Line a shallow 7 x 11 inch baking pan with parchment paper.

- Beat together the sunflower spread, granulated sugar, eggs, and flour until soft and creamy. Spoon the mixture into the pan, spread the surface level, and bake in a preheated oven, at 375°F, for 20 minutes, until golden and just firm to the touch.

- Mix together the confectioners' sugar and lemon juice to make a smooth, runny icing, then drizzle over the cake with a teaspoon.

- Cut into 12 squares or fingers and pile a few soft candies on top of each.

 Penny Candy Squares

Cut a loaf pound cake into 1 inch cubes. Melt 3 tablespoons lemon curd with 1 tablespoon water in a saucepan and stir until smooth. Brush the lemon curd over the cubes, then roll in dried flaked coconut. Top with a few soft candies.

 Penny Candy "Pizza"

Unroll 1 sheets store-bought rolled dough pie crust and cut out the largest circle you can, using a plate as a guide. Place on a baking sheet and bake in a preheated oven, at 400°F, for 10 minutes, until golden. Spread with 3 tablespoons lemon curd and sprinkle chopped fruit and mixed soft candies, such as gumdrops and jelly candies, over the top.

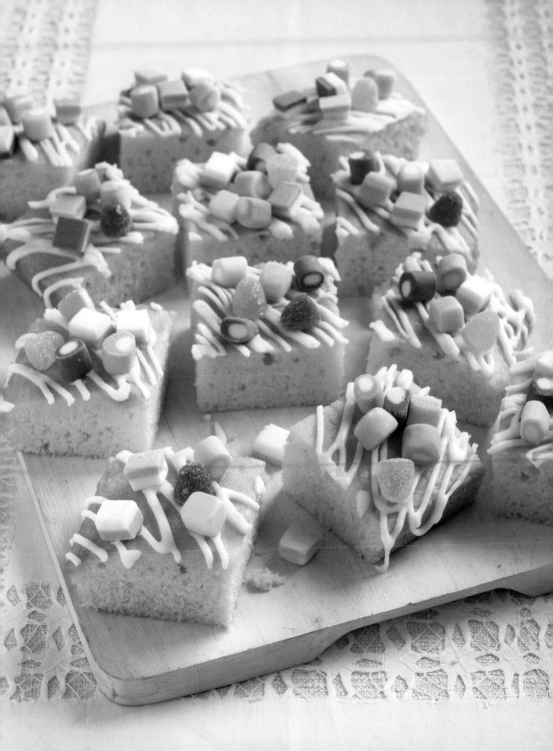

Index

Page references in *italics* indicate photographs

Acknowledgments

Recipes **Emma Jane Frost**
Executive Editor **Eleanor Maxfield**
Editor **Jo Wilson**
Copy Editor **Alison Copland**
Art Direction **Tracy Killick & Geoff Fennell for Tracy Killick Art Direction and Design**
Original Design Concept **www.gradedesign.com**
Designer **Geoff Fennell for Tracy Killick Art Direction and Design**
Photographer **William Reavell**
Home Economist **Emma Jane Frost**
Prop Stylist **Liz Hippisley**
Production Controller **Davide Pontiroli**